The Human face

Overleaf
*A montage from printed
ephemera by Gwyther Irwin*

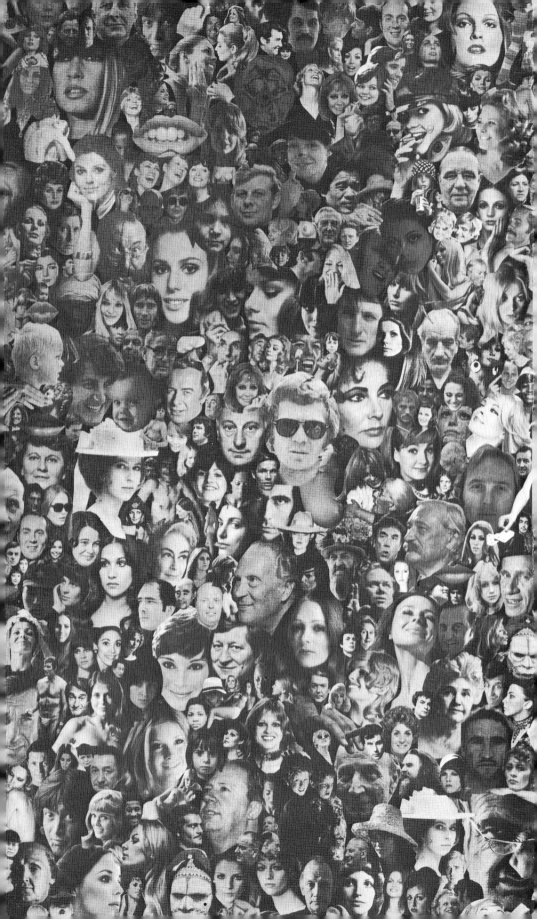

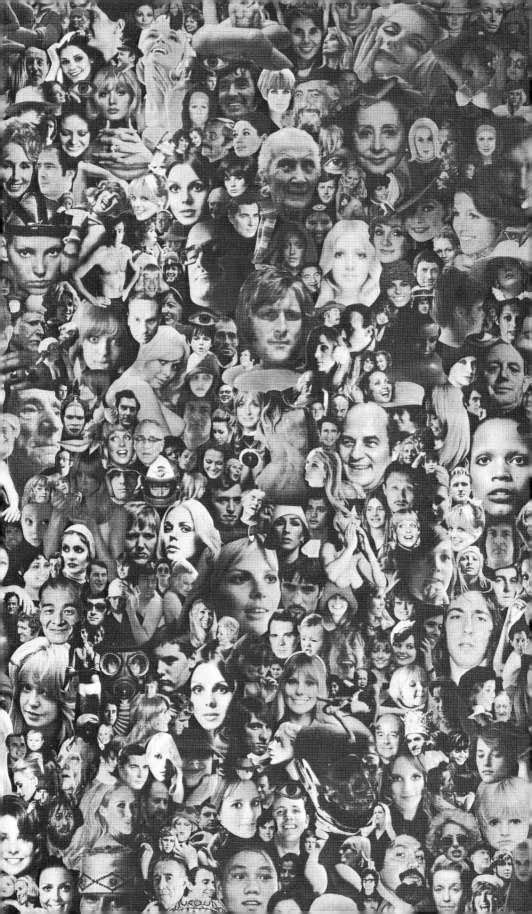

John Liggett   Constable, London

The human face

*First published in 1974
by Constable &
Company Limited
10 Orange Street
London WC2H 7EG*

*Copyright © 1974 by
John Liggett*

*Book designer &
Art Editor
Graham Bishop*

*Filmset and printed in
Great Britain by
BAS Printers Limited,
Wallop, Hampshire*

SBN 09 458170 3

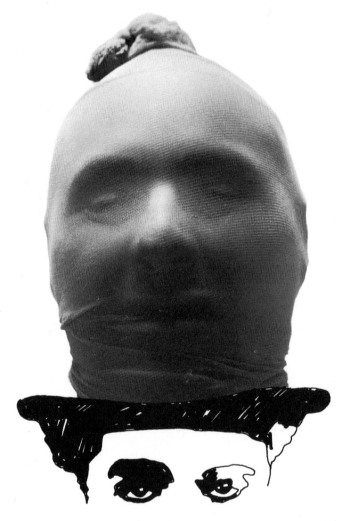

To Arline

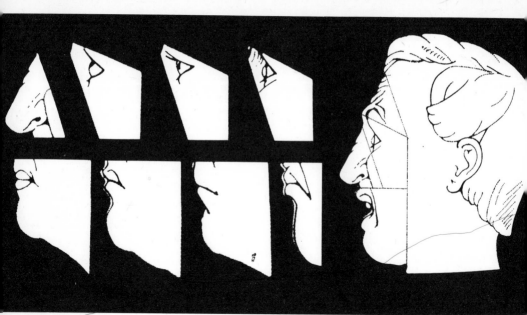

A model for the demonstration of facial expression. Piderit features from Boring and Titchener, 1923

Acknowledgements **x**
Illustrations **xi**
1 Skin and bone **2**
2 Sex, age and race **20**
3 Primitive elaboration **42**
4 Sophisticated elaboration **60**
5 Frames for the face **80**
6 Artful concealment **110**
7 Changing the structure **124**
8 Beauty **138**
9 The face in the mind **158**
10 Guides to character? **180**
11 Features and temperaments **216**
12 Health and disease **232**
13 Occupational faces **240**
14 The art of judgement **258**
Index **283**

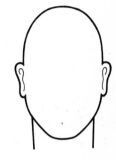

Acknowledgements In writing this book I have made use of a great number of sources and illustrations, many of which are acknowledged in the text or in the list of illustrations. I should, however, like to express my gratitude to the following: to the helpful staffs of UNESCO, the Musée de l'Homme, Illustration Research Service, The Wellcome Museum of the History of Medicine and of both City and University College Libraries in Cardiff, to Colin Voisey, Head of Film Department, H.T.V., Wales, and to my good friend Dr. R. Philip Williams for his valuable comments on the text.

Above all, I would like to acknowledge the immeasurable debt of gratitude I owe to my wife, Arline, for her many original ideas, for her tireless research and discussion, and for her unfailing stimulation, support and encouragement all of which have made this book possible.

University College, Cardiff. 1974

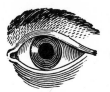

Frontispiece/ Gwyther Irwin

Charlie Chaplin/stocking mask **vi**

Piderit composite **viii**

Chap. **1** Embryos **1** *Human Embryology* Hamilton *et al*

Primitive skulls **2** The Trustees of the British
   Natural History Museum

Reconstructed heads **2** The Trustees of the
   British Natural History Museum

Pericles **6** Folke Henschen *The Human Skull*

Erasmus **6** After Folke Henschen *The Human Skull*

Phrenological bust **7**

Muscle effects **9** After Duval *Anatomy for Artists*

Muscle diagrams **10**

Muscle diagram **11**

Skin: cross section **12**

Skin elasticity **13** Corry Bevington

Ebony and *Focus* advertisements **15** Courtesy of
   Keystone Laboratories and Outdoor Girl
   Cosmetics Ltd.

Facial asymmetry **17** Graham Bishop

Lincoln mosaic **19** Courtesy of L. D. Harmon and
   Bell Telephone Laboratories, USA

Lincoln engraving **19**

Chap. **2** European model **20** Courtesy of Elizabeth Arden

Milanese centenarian **20** Popperfoto

Wagogo native **20** Popperfoto

Dark female eye **22** Graham Bishop

Passive impression **22** Graham Bishop

Changes in proportions with age **24** after
   Krukenberg *Der Gesichtsausdrück des Menschen*

Wrinkles of old age **25** Courtesy of UNESCO/Gerda
   Bohm

Baby's face **25** Anthea Sieveking

Crow's feet **25** Corry Bevington

W. H. Auden **26** *The Times*

David Frost **27** Godfrey Argent

Jack Benny **27** Universal Pictorial Press

Negroid face **30** Graham Bishop

Mongoloid face **30** Musée de l'Homme

Arab face **30** Courtesy of UNESCO/Hohm

Caucasoid face **31** Popperfoto

Chap. 2   Modern Indian faces **32** Contemporary Films
African face **32** Corry Bevington
American Indian face **33** Philadelphia Museum of
    Art/A. J. Wyatt
Negro face **34** Contemporary Films/Carillon
European face **34** Popperfoto
Arab face **34** Courtesy of UNESCO/Paul Almasy
Negro girl **36** Courtesy of UNESCO/Pittet
Mixed characteristics **40** John Liggett
Nationality undetectable **41** Courtesy of UNESCO/
    Pittet

Chap. 3   African girl **42** Courtesy of Musée de l'Homme
African woman **44** Courtesy of John Hillaby
Nefertiti **45** (a) Wellcome Institute of the History
    of Medicine
Nefertiti in profile **45** (b) Mansell Collection
Amarna Princess **45** Folke Henschen *The Human
    Skull*
Head deformation, modern **46** Folke Henschen
    The Human Skull
Artificially deformed head **46** Folke Henschen
    The Human Skull
Devices for deformation **47** Folke Henschen
    The Human Skull
Congolese woman **47** Courtesy of Musée de
    l'Homme
Ear deformation **48** Courtesy of Pitt Rivers
    Museum
Mouth deformation **49** Courtesy of Musée de
    l'Homme
Mouth deformation **49** Courtesy of Musée de
    l'Homme
Mouth deformation **49** Courtesy of Pitt Rivers
    Museum
Ear deformation **49** Courtesy of UNESCO
Ear ornamentation **49** Courtesy of Pitt Rivers
    Museum
Ear deformation **49** Courtesy of Pitt Rivers
    Museum
Nose deformation **49** Courtesy of Musée de
    l'Homme

Chap. 3   Mouth-piercing **49** Courtesy of UNESCO/
  Labordère, 1965
Teeth-filing **50** Courtesy of Musée de l'Homme
Scarification **53** Courtesy of UNESCO/Pittet, 1962
Cicatrisation **53** Courtesy of Musée de l'Homme
Tattooing, South America **57** Courtesy of Musée
  de l'Homme
Tattooing, Japan **57** Courtesy of Musée de
  l'Homme
Tattooing, Maoris **57** Courtesy of Musée de
  l'Homme
Tattooing, Europe **58** Popperfoto

Chap. 4   Roman cosmetic jar **60**
Roman period facial model **62** The Trustees of the
  British Museum
Kohl tubes **63/64** The Trustees of the British
  Museum
Double kohl tube **64** The Trustees of the British
  Museum
Egyptian eye-paint boxes **64** Radio Times Hulton
An Egyptian lady **64** Radio Times Hulton
Unguent and eye-paint jars **64** The Trustees of the
  British Museum
Indian woman **65** The Trustees of the Victoria
  and Albert Museum
Willcotes Effigies **65** Mansell Collection
(a) Burgundian lady **66** Mansell Collection
(b) Mediaeval lady **66** The Trustees of the
  National Gallery
(c) Florentine lady **66** The Trustees of the
  National Gallery
Glenda Jackson **66** BBC photograph
Maria Gunning **68** The Trustees of the Courtauld
  Institute and The Tate Gallery
Louis xvth and xvith toilet articles **70** Popperfoto
Madame de Pompadour **71** The Trustees of the
  National Galleries of Scotland
Madame du Barry **71** The Trustees of the British
  Museum
Madame de Pompadour **71** The Mansell Collection
Marie Antoinette **71** The Mansell Collection

Chap. 4 Pears' advertisement **72** *The Graphic* 1889
Victorian engravings **73**
Beauty School, USA **74** Popperfoto
Facial massage **74** Popperfoto
Mud pack **74** Popperfoto
Cosmetic aids **74**
Cosmetic aids **75**
Modern eye decoration **76**
Modern eye decoration **77**
Eye make-up **78**
Party make-up **78** André Carrara
Gary Glitter **79** Camera Press London
Chap. 5 Two faces **80** Graham Bishop
Facial trimmings **81** Corry Bevington
Nomad woman, Upper Nigeria **81** Corry Bevington
Bamako student **81** Courtesy UNESCO/A. Tessore
Nigerian sign **82** Corry Bevington
The Brush **82** Courtesy of Vidal Sassoon. Photo:
    Barry Lategan. Model: Christine Walton
The V.S. Cut **82** Courtesy of Vidal Sassoon
The Thatch **82** Courtesy of Vidal Sassoon. Photo:
    Barry Lategan. Model: Nell Campbell
Hair styling **83** Courtesy of Helena Rubinstein
Male styles **83** Courtesy of Vidal Sassoon
Isadora **83** Courtesy of Vidal Sassoon
The Fall **83** Courtesy of Vidal Sassoon. Photo:
    Patrick Hunt. Model: Moyra Swan
Nubians **84** The Trustees of the British Museum
Venetian fashions **84** Bruhn and Tilke *A Pictorial
    History of Costume*
16th century lady **84** The Trustees of the National
    Portrait Gallery
Greek Apollo **85** Mansell Collection
Charles II **86** The Trustees of the Victoria and
    Albert Museum
Duchess of Richmond **86** Dean and Chapter of
    Westminster Abbey
18th century bonnets **86** The Trustees of the
    Victoria and Albert Museum
Lady, 1761 **86** The Trustees of the Victoria and
    Albert Museum

Chap. 5   Cromwellian styling **87** The Trustees of the
            National Portrait Gallery

Lady, 1780 **88** Radio Times Hulton

Social caricatures of 18th century hair styling **89**
    Radio Times Hulton

Wig designs **92** Wendy Cooper *Hair*

Mr Speaker **93** *The Times*. Courtesy of The
    Speaker

Wigs by Vidal Sassoon **94/95** Courtesy of Vidal
    Sassoon

Baldness **95** Concealing baldness **95** Malcolm
    Pendrill Ltd. Photo. Courtesy of Wig Artists

Stone relief **96** The Trustees of the British Museum

Medusa mask **96** The Trustees of the Warburg
    Institute

Sargon **96** Directorate General of Antiquities, Iraq

Bearded Bacchus **96**

Amun-Re **97** The Trustees of the British Museum

Henry VIII **99** The Trustees of the National
    Portrait Gallery

Beards and moustaches **101** The Trustees of the
    Victoria and Albert Museum

Naval beard **102** The Trustees of the Victoria and
    Albert Museum

Longfellow **102** The Trustees of the Victoria and
    Albert Museum

Seventies style **102** Courtesy of Vidal Sassoon

Adolph Hitler **102** *The Times*

Mark Twain **103** The Trustees of the Victoria and
    Albert Museum

Moustache advertisement **103** Mary Evans Picture
    Library (Wendy Cooper *Hair*)

Charlie Chaplin **103**

Diplomatic Corps Marshal **104** Universal
    Pictorial Press

The Homburg **104** Courtesy G. A. Dunn and Co.

The cloth cap **104**

Gainsborough Lady **105** The Trustees of the
    National Gallery

Edwardian millinery **106/107** Radio Times
    Hulton

Chap. 5   Millinery of the seventies **106/107** 5·57/64:
Graham Bishop 5·59/63: Courtesy of Helena
Rubinstein
Turban **108** Corry Bevington
Straw hats **108** Corry Bevington
Nagasaki lady **109** Arnoldus Montanus *Ambassades
Memorables*

Chap. 6   Fancy-dress mask **110** Graham Bishop
Bicycling mask **110** from *L'Illustration*, 1903
Winter mask **110** The Trustees of the Victoria and
Albert Museum
Incognito **111** The Trustees of the Victoria and
Albert Museum
Masks, 17th century **112** John Bulwer *The
Artificial Changeling*, 1654
Turkish woman **112** Cesare Vecellio *De gli habiti
antichi*
18th century mask **112** The Trustees of the
British Museum
Automobile wear **112** from *L'Illustration*, 1903
Veil, 70's **113** Graham Bishop
Filipino fishermen **114** Camera Press London.
Feast-day costume, Algeria **114** UNESCO/Lajoux,
1961
Indian woman in purdah **115** UNESCO/ J.
Bhownagary, 1952
Young bride, Tripoli **115** Radio Times Hulton
Afghanistan housewives **115** UNESCO/Cart, 1963
Concert **117** The Trustees of the City Art Gallery,
Manchester
French fan **117** The Trustees of the Victoria and
Albert Museum
Quizzing glass **118** Radio Times Hulton
Spectacle Shop **118** The Trustees of the Victoria
and Albert Museum
Sun visor **119** Graham Bishop
Spectacles **119** Courtesy Mary Quant
Artificial Changeling **120** John Bulwer *The
Artificial Changeling*, 1654
Face patches, France **120** The Trustees of the
Victoria and Albert Museum

Chap. 6   Patches, 1973 **123** Graham Bishop
Chap. 7   Tagliacozzi **124** The University Library, Bologna
Damaged nose **127** Radio Times Hulton
Hypertelorism **127** Daily Telegraph Colour Library
Ear surgery **127** Courtesy Leslie Gardiner *Faces,*
    Figures and Feelings
Nasal proportions **129** The Trustees of the
    British Museum
Tom Jones **130** Popperfoto
Nose surgery **130** Radio Times Hulton
Rhinoplasty **130** Radio Times Hulton
Nose operation **131** The Sunday Times
Chin-line **132** Courtesy of Leslie E. Gardiner
    Faces, Figures and Feelings
Surgery for eyelid pouches **133** Courtesy of Leslie
    E. Gardiner *Faces, Figures and Feelings*
Chap. 8   Perfect proportions **138** The Mansell Collection
Head of Venus **139** The Trustees of the National
    Gallery
Facial proportions **140** By gracious permission of
    Her Majesty the Queen
Hogarth **141** The Trustees of the National
    Portrait Gallery
The Uglies **141** Topix photo. Peter Dunne
Criteria of beauty **143** from Curry, Brislin, Liggett
An ideal of the seventies **145** Courtesy Helena
    Rubenstein
Monroe **147** National Film Archive
Ekland **148** National Film Archive
Gable **149** National Film Archive
Vietnamese **149** UNESCO/Lajoux
Victorian ideals **153** The Trustees of The Tate
    Gallery
Picasso **154** The Trustees of The Tate Gallery
David Hume **155** The Trustees of the National
    Portrait Gallery of Scotland
Garbo **157** National Film Archive
Chap. 9   Nude **158** Jeanloup Sieff
Forehead **158** Graham Bishop
Naked peoples **158** National Museum of
    Ethnology, Leiden, Holland

Chap. 9   Signals during lovemaking **160** Graham Bishop
Bowl made from skull **162** The Trustees of the
Victoria and Albert Museum
Shrunken heads **162** Courtesy of Musée de
l'Homme
Mummified head **163** Courtesy of Musée de
l'Homme
Widow with husband's skull **163** Popperfoto
Nigerian mask **164** The Trustees of the Pitt Rivers
Museum
Ambiguous masks **164** The Trustees of the Pitt
Rivers Museum
Ambiguous mask from New Ireland **164**
Congolese mask **164** The Trustees of the British
Museum
Tutankhamun **167** Graham Bishop
Mycaenaean funerary mask **167** Himar Fotoarchiv
'No' masks **168** The Trustees of the Pitt Rivers
Museum
Ceylon devil-dancer's mask **168** The Trustees of
the British Museum
Ceylon mask for curing stammering **168** The
Trustees of the British Museum
Javanese mask **168** The Trustees of the British
Museum
Wooden mask of Ceylon **169** The Trustees of the
British Museum
Clown face **170** Robert Wood *Victorian Delights*
Japanese mask **171** Courtesy of Musée de l'Homme
Face and torso **174/176** The author
Facial imagery in architecture **175** Courtesy of the
Italian State Tourist Office
Mask evoking body imagery **176** Courtesy of
Musée de l'Homme
Magritte **177** Collection George Melly, London.
© by ADAGP Paris 1973
Venus of Willendorf **178** Graham Bishop
Grotesque **178** The Trustees of the Victoria and
Albert Museum
Ivory engraving **178** R. Schmidt *Dawn of the
Human Mind*

Chap. 9   Face and body imagery **179** Division of Photography, Chicago Field Museum of Natural
History

Chap. 10   A guide to character **180** Octavius Hill

Astrological guides **183** Cardarno *Fisionomia
Astrologica*

Podoscopy **184**

The temperaments **185** George Combe *System of
Phrenology*

Goat-faced men **186** J. B. Della Porta *Of Celestial
Physiognomy,* 1627

J. B. Della Porta **187**

Lavater **188-198, 202/203** J. K. Lavater *Essays in
Physiognomy,* 1765

Silhouette of Lavater **200**

Socrates **203**

Bust by Fowler **207** The Trustees of the Wellcome
Institute

Bust by Spurzheim **207** Courtesy of Musée de
l'Homme

Incognito **207** The Trustees of the British Museum

Craniology cartoon **208** The Trustees of the
British Museum

Phrenological drawings and 'Should we marry?'
advertisement **210/211** George Combe *A System
of Phrenology,* p. 210. From *Psychology Today,* **211**

Darwin **214** The President and Council of the
Royal College of Surgeons of England

Chap. 11   Aristotle **216** Mansell Collection

Line drawings from books by Lavater, Simms and
Wells **218-230**

Eight grotesque heads **225** By gracious permission
of Her Majesty the Queen

Faces test **226** John Liggett *Faces test*

General Wolfe **231** The Trustees of the National
Portrait Gallery

Racial determination **231** Radio Times Hulton

Chap. 12   Facies hippocratica **232** adapted from Bellak *The
Face in Medicine*

Saddle nose of syphilis **234** Courtesy of the
Wellcome Museum

Chap. 12   Exophthalmic goitre **235** Thorek *Modern Surgical Techniques*. Courtesy of The Wellcome Museum Montgomery *Clinical Endocrinology for Surgeons* **235**

Cushing's Disease **236/7** Williams *Textbook of Endocrinology*. Courtesy of The Wellcome Museum Acromegaly **238/9** Courtesy of The Wellcome Museum

Chap. 13   Composite photograph

Henrik Ibsen **247** Courtesy Royal Norwegian Embassy

F. M. Dostoyevsky **247** Novosti Press Agency

Hans Christian Andersen **247** Courtesy Royal Danish Embassy

John Ruskin **247** The Trustees of the Victoria and Albert Museum

Chas. L. Dodgson **247** Radio Times Hulton

M. K. Gandhi **247** Radio Times Hulton

David Livingstone **248**

Ralph W. Emerson **248** Radio Times Hulton

Johannes V. Jensen **248** Courtesy Royal Danish Ministry for Foreign Affairs

Richard Burton **248** The Trustees of the Victoria and Albert Museum

Andrew Carnegie **248** Radio Times Hulton

Henry Ford **248** Radio Times Hulton

King Frederik **249** Courtesy Royal Danish Ministry for Foreign Affairs

King Olav V **249** Courtesy Royal Norwegian Embassy

Gregor Mendel **249** Courtesy Moravian Museum, Brno

Edward Fitzgerald **249** The Trustees of the Victoria and Albert Museum

L. Tolstoi **249** Novosti Press Agency

Lord Rutherford **249** The Trustees of the National Gallery

M. Gorki **250** Novosti Press Agency

A. P. Chekhov **250** Novosti Press Agency

Kandinsky **250** Courtesy of Marlborough Fine Art

T. S. Eliot **250** Angus McBean

Chap. 13 Herbert Morrison **250** Central Office of
Information

Sidney Webb **250** The Trustees of the Victoria
and Albert Museum

William Gladstone **251** The Trustees of the
Victoria and Albert Museum

George Cadbury **251** Radio Times Hulton

Andrew Mellon **251** Radio Times Hulton

N. A. Rimsky-Korsakov **251** Novosti Press
Agency

Ralph Vaughan Williams **251** BBC

Carl Nielsen **251** Courtesy Royal Danish Embassy

John D. Rockefeller **252** Radio Times Hulton

Marshal Pétain **252**

Robert E. Lee **252** Radio Times Hulton

General Patton **252** Imperial War Museum

William Richard Morris (Lord Nuffield) **252** Radio
Times Hulton

S. Prokofiev **252** Novosti Press Agency

S. Shostakovich **253** Novosti Press Agency

Sir Alexander Fleming **253** Central Office of
Information

Sir John Cockcroft **253** Central Office of
Information

C. E. M. Joad **253** Radio Times Hulton

A. Khachaturyan **253** Novosti Press Agency

Benjamin Britten **253** Universal Pictorial Press

U Thant **254** Courtesy of United Nations

Field-Marshal Alexander **254** Keystone Press
Agency

Dag Hammarskjold **254** Courtesy of United
Nations

Chap. 14 Emotion **258**

Duchenne's experiments **260** Duchenne *Mecanisme
de la Physionomie Humaine*

Emotional face **260**

Emotional face **261**

Couples in love **262** BBC

Emotional face **263**

Emotional face **264**

Couples in love **265** BBC

Chap. **14**   Emotional faces **267** Keystone Press Agency

Rudolph's drawings **269** Rudolph *Der Ausdruck der Gemütsbewegungen des Menschen*

Eyes and eyebrows **270** Adapted from photo. Courtesy Air Express

'True' series **276** Courtesy Colin Voisey, Harlech Television. Photo. Ivor Jacobs

'False' series **276** Courtesy Colin Voisey, Harlech Television. Photo. Ivor Jacobs

'True' series **280**

'True' series **280**

'False' series **280**

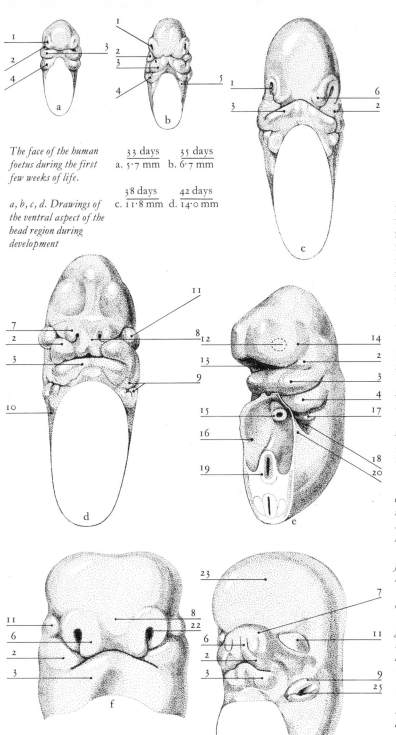

The face of the human foetus during the first few weeks of life.

a, b, c, d. Drawings of the ventral aspect of the head region during development

33 days
a. 5·7 mm

35 days
b. 6·7 mm

38 days
c. 11·8 mm

42 days
d. 14·0 mm

1 Olfactory pit
2 Maxillary process
3 Mandibular process
4 Hyoid arch
5 Third pharyngeal arch
6 Medial nasal process
7 Lateral nasal process
8 Fronto-nasal process
9 Pinna
10 Cervical sinus
11 Eye
12 Nasal placode
13 Stomatodaeum
14 Lens placode
15 Bulbus cordis
16 Pericardial cavity
17 Third pharyngeal arch
18 Fourth pharyngeal arch
19 Foregut
20 Epi-pericardial ridge
21 Spinal cord
22 Primitive ant. naris
23 Forebrain
24 Epithelial plug
25 External auditory meatus

e Drawing of the left ventro-lateral aspect of the head end of a 16 mm human embryo 35 days

f Drawing of the ventral aspect of the face of a 10·0 mm human embryo 37 days

g Drawing of the left ventro-lateral aspect of a model of the head of an 18·0 mm human embryo 50 days
Drawings (after Streeter) a, b, c and d are of a different scale from e, f and g
Overall foetal lengths are given

I

I Skin and bone

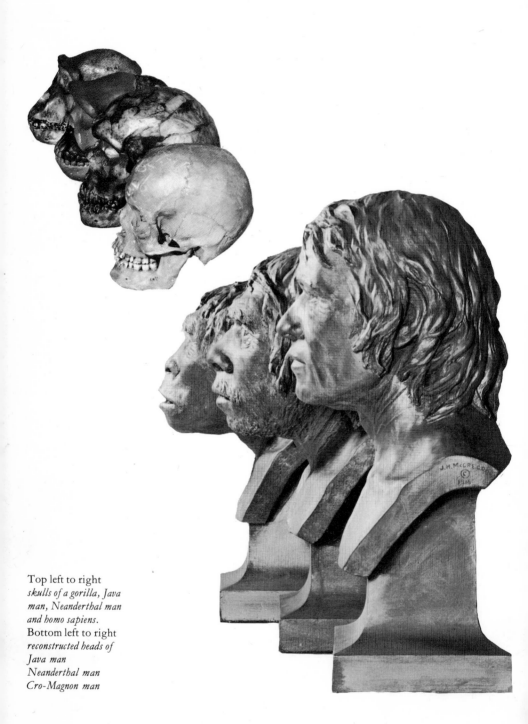

Top left to right
*skulls of a gorilla, Java
man, Neanderthal man
and homo sapiens.*
Bottom left to right
*reconstructed heads of
Java man
Neanderthal man
Cro-Magnon man*

Every human embryo passes through a stage during the
fifth week of life when it has clearly-marked fish-like gills.
These gills are a reminder of the time, millions of years ago,
when man's remote ancestors were sea-dwellers. The story
of the face really begins about four hundred million years
ago when some of the more intelligent and adventurous of
these sea creatures began to stray on to dry land. To survive
out of water they needed an entirely new kind of breathing
equipment; it was no longer possible to secure oxygen by
the old method of pumping great quantities of oxygenated
water through their fish gills. So lungs began to evolve and
the old fish gills began to disappear—or rather, because this
is the way of evolution, to change into something else.
First the bones of the gill arches began to evolve slowly into
jaw bones. And then the gill muscles, originally used for
pumping water, gradually became transformed into a new
kind of muscular veil across the front of the skull. It was
this muscular veil which was eventually to become the
human face.

The story of the evolution of the face is one of great
variety: variety not only in the shapes and proportions of its
underlying support, the skull, but also in the muscles and
skin which provide its covering. The face, and its bony
framework the skull, have changed a great deal even in
comparatively recent geological times. The illustration
shows three important stages in the development of the
skulls of early man—from the most primitive 'Java Man',
through 'Neanderthal Man', to the relatively recent 'Cro-
Magnon Man'. If we examine these skulls closely we find
some striking similarities with man's cousins, the anthropoid
apes: for example, the prominent 'superciliary ridge' above
the eyes, whose purpose was to strengthen the brow to
withstand the enormous forces exerted by the powerful jaw
muscles used in the primeval forest for tearing and chewing.
As primitive man learned to climb trees, and so became
increasingly dexterous, he began to break up his food with
his hands—and the jaw and the brow ridge gradually became less prominent. He still needed some leverage, however, to chew his food—and so there evolved that uniquely
human characteristic, the chin. At the same time as the jaws
became smaller and less powerful, the prominent super-

ciliary ridge also began to disappear, and man's forehead bones became smoother. Indeed, the whole of the front of the face became steeper as the prognathous jaw receded and the forehead moved forward. The zoologist Camper, who, two centuries ago, first noticed this gradual change in the 'facial angle', believed that the steepness of the face was a valuable guide to a skull's level of evolutionary sophistication.

There are several important respects, however, in which the skulls of primitive men differed from those of the apes. Whereas apes tend to be broad-headed or 'brachycephalic' most of the 'Fossil Men' so far unearthed have had longer, narrower, 'dolichocephalic' skulls.

There is enormous variety to be found even today in the shapes and proportions of the faces of modern man. Not only are there great contrasts between the races—there are also great variations *within* each racial group. It is just as difficult to find two identical Negro faces as it is to find two similar Caucasians. The human face is, without question, man's most varied—as well as his most variable—attribute.

There are no less than fourteen different bones supporting and underlying the face, and the shapes and sizes of these vary a great deal from person to person. Some of them change markedly during a lifetime. One of the more conspicuous of these changes is the shrinkage or 'resorption' of the jawbone which sometimes occurs in old age after the teeth are lost. During childhood, too, there are some striking changes in some of the facial bones—such as those of the cheeks. In babyhood these are extremely shallow; the distance from nostrils to eyes is very much smaller than it 'should be' according to adult proportions. The baby's cranium, by contrast, is proportionally very large. It is these two factors acting together—large forehead and shallow cheeks—which produce the characteristic 'baby-face'.

There is, broadly speaking, a correspondence between skull size and body size—the head usually being, at maturity, about one-seventh of the total body height, though it may occupy a considerably higher fraction in infancy: the head of the newborn baby may be as much as one-fifth of its body length. But it is not just age which affects the proportions of the head and face: sex, too, is an important factor. Female skulls are in general only four-fifths the size of those of males—a difference, incidentally, which does not confer any superiority of intelligence on the male. The male usually has a larger and wider jaw, and often, too, a slight prominence above the brow (a relic perhaps of the old superciliary arch), known as the glabellar eminence.

The overall size of faces and skulls varies a great deal. Lenin's skull, for example, was very large—as was that of Swedenborg, which was unusually 'keel-shaped', or 'scapho-cephalic'—excessively long and narrow when viewed from above. Plutarch tells that the great Athenian Pericles was called 'onion-head' by his contemporaries and that he required a special helmet to cover his unusual 'peak skull'. Several of the world's great novelists seem to have been afflicted with disproportionately large faces and heads—especially when young. Mark Twain was once described as a youngster 'with a huge head and an ink-smudged face', and Thomas Hardy, whilst still at school, as 'the littlest fellow with the biggest head in class'. He was, it is said, a weak, puny child, a 'little fellow with the face of an old man'. The artist Toulouse-Lautrec also had an abnormally large head and face.

Lest we draw premature conclusions about head size and brilliance, however, let it be said right away that there have been many great scholars with remarkably *small* heads. Erasmus had a peculiarly short, 'hyperbrachycephalic' head, and a very small brain, estimated as probably no more than 1160 grams in weight (an ordinary brain weighs about 1400 grams). He wore a specially-constructed wig and a large biretta hat to disguise his tiny head. Anatole France, too, had an unusually small head. And the great German anatomist Roux was so worried about his dismally tiny head that he ordered from his deathbed that his brain be removed and destroyed as soon as he was dead—for fear that it would otherwise be preserved as an anatomical curiosity. There are many more examples of brilliant men with small brains, and it is now quite clear that there is little relationship between head or brain-size and intelligence in man.

But there was a time, nonetheless, in the early nineteenth century, when there was an almost frenzied interest in the

Pericles was known as
'onion-head' to his
contemporaries on
account of his dispro-
portionately tall head
and domed, 'peak-skull'.
In nearly all his statues
he is seen wearing a
helmet which, according
to Plutarch, the sculptors
used to conceal these
'blemishes'

Erasmus (1466–1536)
was notoriously vain
and always concealed his
exceptionally small
head with his large
biretta. He never
appeared in public
without it

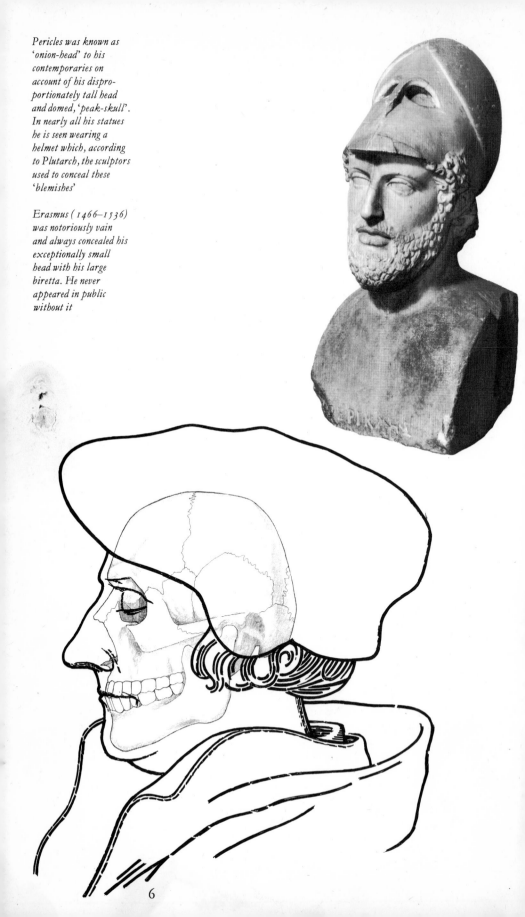

skull among ordinary men and women. It was not so much its size as the curves and bumps on its surface which excited their interest, for these curves and bumps were popularly believed to be an infallible guide to personality, character and ability. The 'phrenologists' Gall and Spurzheim had somehow managed to convince their contemporaries that a man's talents and weaknesses could be 'read' by feeling his head, because, as they declared, each bump was caused by a particularly well-developed part of the brain lying under the skull. And each different mental 'faculty' had its own special area; a strong sense of 'foresight', for example, would be revealed by a bump at the top of the centre of the face at the hairline. Modern research has made it clear that these old phrenological ideas were quite mistaken; particular mental qualities do *not* result from strong growth of particular parts of the brain neither are they reflected by bumps on the head's surface.

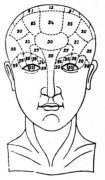

In the mid-19th century, many people believed that the shape of the skull both affected, and indicated, a person's temperament

The great and abiding interest of the human face derives as much from its mobility—its remarkable powers of expression—as from its shape. And it is the facial musculature which makes this possible. There are more than a hundred different muscles lying just below the surface of the face. These lie in many different directions, criss-crossing each other in a thousand different ways, making possible a rich variety of complex, subtle and beautiful movements. Many of the muscles are anchored at one end to the skull. This means that when the muscle contracts in response to a message from the brain, the unattached end is pulled closer to the end attached to the skull so that the skin and tissues lying on top of the muscle will also be made to move at the same time. The corner of the mouth, for example, may be pulled upwards into a smiling position. The main muscles of the face are illustrated overleaf. Some of them have acquired popular names as well as standard anatomical descriptions. The *frontalis,* for instance, is sometimes called 'the muscle of attention'. This has the effect of lifting up the eyebrows, also of helping to pull the eyes wide open. But it is frequently involved, too, in more complex movements of the face—such as those which occur in 'puzzlement' or 'uncertainty'. In both of these expressions, however, yet another muscle is simultaneously involved: the *supraorbital orbicular,* popularly called the 'muscle of reflection'. This reminds us that most of our facial expressions are, in fact, brought about by the simultaneous action of many muscles.

The skin itself is separated from the muscles by a layer of fatty tissue which may be thick or thin, smooth or corrugated, according to age, sex and constitution. There are several important cushions of fat lying just below the skin of the face which exert a profound effect on facial appearance. An example of one of these is to be found at the root of the nose between the eyes, another between the nose and the upper lip. Yet another can be felt at the point of the chin. Some of these fatty cushions vary a great deal during lifetime. When babies are very young, for example, their cheeks are puffed out with 'sucking-pads' between their *masseter* and *buccinator* muscles, which serve to support the cheeks during feeding. The importance of these sucking pads in nature's scheme is indicated by their presence even in starving and emaciated children.

The appearance of the skin depends on several factors—its texture, its thickness, the nature of the blood circulation, and the characteristics of the tissues beneath the skin. Its appearance, too, depends very much on its flexibility, whether it happens to be pulled taut or has, with age or disease, wrinkled and lost its elasticity. Its thickness varies considerably in different parts of the face: on the eyelids, for example, it is very thin, though not so thin as on the lips, where it is so transparent that the colour of the flesh beneath can be seen. The thickness of the skin, indeed, affects its colour: where it is thin it tends to be pink and where it is thick rather more yellow.

The lustre and transparency of the skin varies a great deal in different individuals, the skin being thinner, smoother and more transparent in females than in males. There are differences, too, in the tissues supporting it—in females there is usually more underlying fatty tissue, in youth at least, which gives it its characteristically smooth appearance. The loss of this fatty support in middle age may produce wrinkling because the skin and its underlay may shrink at different rates. A further cause of wrinkling is that the skin often loses the elasticity of youth and so cannot adjust as once it could even to the more limited expansion and con-

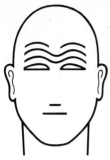

1 frontalis
Attention/
Astonishment

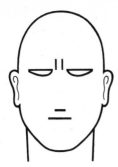

2 orbicularis oculi
Reflection/Meditation

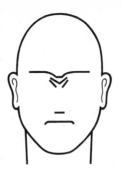

3 procerus
Harshness
Menace
Aggression

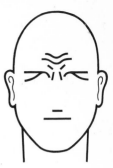

4 corrugator
Sorrow

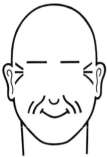

5 zygomaticus major
Laughter

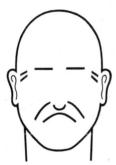

6 levator labii
superioris et alae
nasi
Discontent/Grief

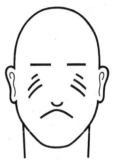

7 levator labii
Extreme grief with
tears

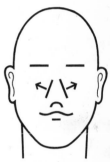

8 compressor naris
Attention/
Sensuousness

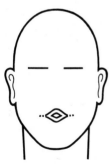

9 orbicularis oris
Pouting or pulling-in
(biting) lips

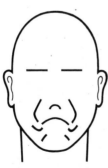

10 depressor anguli
oris
Contempt

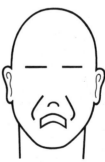

11 depressor labii
inferioris
Disgust

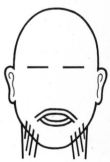

12 platysma
Anger, pain
Torture, Extreme
Exertion

*Some of the more
important facial
muscles concerned in
expression*

1 frontalis
2 orbicularis oculi
3 procerus
4 corrugator
5 zygomaticus major
6 levator labii
   superioris et alae
   nasi
7 levator labii
8 compressor naris
9 orbicularis oris
10 depressor anguli
   oris
11 depressor labii
   inferioris
12 platysma

a zygomaticus
   minor
b masseter *non-
   expressive*
c buccinator *non-
   expressive*
d temporal *non-
   expressive*

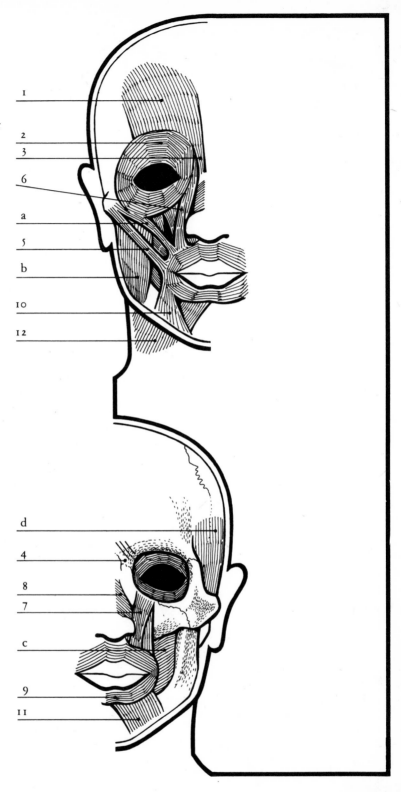

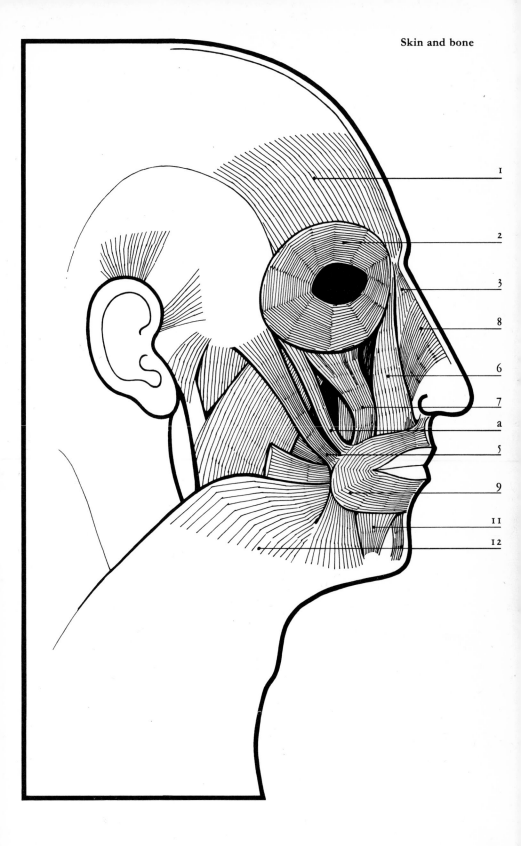

1

2

3

8

6

7

a

5

9

11

12

traction called for by ageing muscles. Lines and wrinkles generally arise at right angles to the direction of the muscles. On the forehead, for example, where the fibres of the underlying *frontalis* muscle lie vertically, the wrinkles tend to develop horizontally. Though wrinkles show great variation both in density and in location, there are some deep furrows or 'rugae' which occur commonly enough to have been given special names. Examples of these are the 'nasolabial' furrows which commonly extend from the outer corners of the nose to the corners of the mouth.

The texture and appearance of the skin of the face owes a great deal to the glands contained within it; these are of two types, sweat glands and sebaceous glands. The latter, which often occur in hair follicles, are more densely distributed on the face and scalp than on any other part of the body. The sebaceous glands are particularly dense on the forehead and nose—and can sometimes render cosmetics difficult to apply. The greasy, oily substance, sebum, secreted by these glands, particularly during adolescence and the early years of sexual maturity, possesses a delicate, but definite and characteristic odour which may serve as a sexual stimulus—at least to those whose noses are young enough to smell it. It is not widely realised that even lightly-perfumed cosmetics may have the effect of completely blanketing this important source of stimulation. In later life, these sebaceous glands tend to become much less active. It is glands of this same general type, incidentally, which secrete the waterproof and insect-proof wax of the ear—and which, in yet another form, secrete the milk from a nursing mother's breast.

The colour of the skin is controlled by inherited factors which follow the genetic laws discovered in the nineteenth century by Mendel. Though only three pairs of genes are involved, it is nonetheless very difficult to predict with certainty what the colour of a new baby of parents of different skin colour is likely to be. The situation is made even more complicated by the fact that 'dark' genes are widely scattered in populations of light peoples. Many anthropologists believe that primitive man was originally coffee-coloured—and that those peoples who moved towards temperate, cloudy regions became adapted to the lack of sunlight by losing, over many generations, their dark

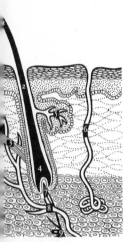

Above *A typical cross section of skin showing:*
1 shaft
2 hair root
3 erector muscle
4 hair bulb
5 sebaceous gland
6 sweat gland
7 papilla
8 blood-vessel
9 nerve

Opposite *The skin's loss of elasticity sometimes becomes very apparent in old age*

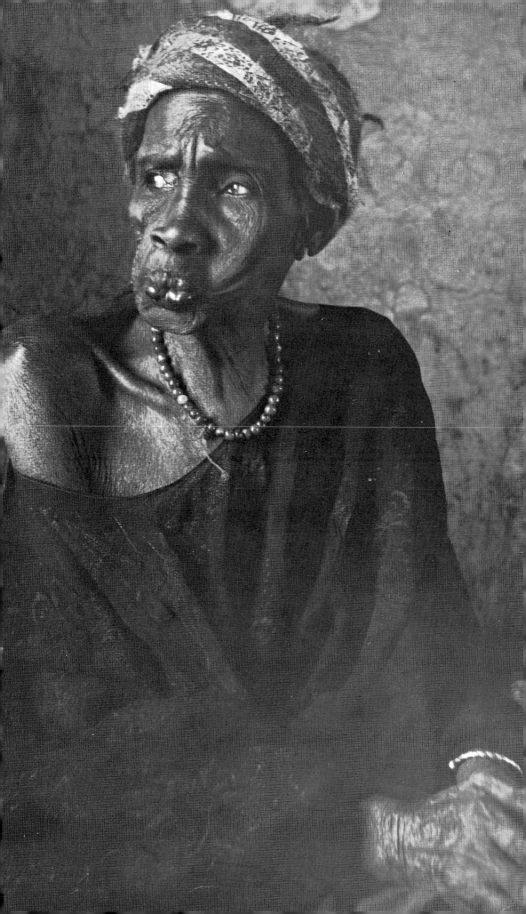

protective pigment, melanin. What little ultraviolet light there was therefore, was able to penetrate their skin to generate the vitamin D essential for health. Of those, on the other hand, who moved towards the tropics, only the fittest—which means the darkest—were able to survive and reproduce.

It is difficult to understand why skin colour should so often provoke such strong emotional reactions. It has sometimes been suggested that an adverse reaction to other skin colours is innate and primitive—even that it might have some biological value, for example, by discouraging people of dissimilar colour from mating and producing unhealthy offspring. But it is now known that exactly the opposite is the case; children of mixed parentage often display 'hybrid vigour'. Furthermore, recent research in America and Britain has made it quite clear that adverse attitudes to skin colours are, in fact, *acquired* during early life from parents and from environmental influences; colour hostility is certainly not inborn. A few minutes' observation of young black and white children playing together makes it quite obvious that they enjoy each other's company and are quite unmoved by their differences in skin colour—if they are even aware of them. Children absorb parental attitudes to colour, as to so many other things, quite unconsciously; no words need be spoken. And such attitudes are much more easily acquired than lost.

To discover just what effect skin colour has on adults' attitudes and behaviour, an American, J. H. Griffin, performed an interesting and courageous experiment in 1959. He took the new drug *Psoralen* and demonstrated first of all that it was possible to stimulate the production of melanin in his skin and so change his colour from white to dark brown. He then moved to a large city in the American deep South and lived for several months as a Negro. He had some highly disturbing experiences—which he relates in his book, *Black Like Me*. A similar experiment was undertaken ten years later by Grace Halsell, a staff writer at the White House. She also took Psoralen pills to darken her skin, disguised her pale eyes with dark contact lenses, and dyed her hair black. She then spent what she described as 'six humiliating months as a black person in the slums of

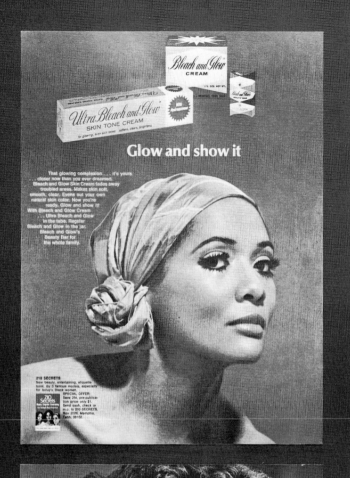

An advertisement from Ebony, *July, 1973* 'The glowing complexion . . . it's yours . . . closer now than you ever dreamed'

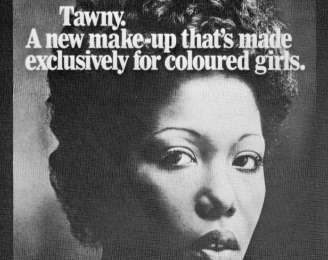

An advertisement from Focus, *July, 1973* 'At last, someone has realised your skin is different.
Not just darker, but different in texture and in its reactions to the ingredients in most cosmetics'

Harlem and Mississippi'—an experience she has recorded in her book, *Soul Sister*. Eventually, by discontinuing treatment with Psoralen, she found she was able to return to her original pale skin colour.

Many other Americans over the past twenty-five years have undertaken the reverse transformation of skin colour—from black to white. Not all, by any means, have done this to avoid the effects of prejudice. The majority have been acting on medical advice to treat a troublesome condition known as *vitiligo,* which disfigures the skin with pale patches. Since dermatologists invariably find it impossible to repigment these pale patches satisfactorily they usually prescribe general bleaching of the whole skin as the best solution. The chemical they use is monobenzylether of hydroquinone (MBEH). The results of such radical transformations from black to white have not always been welcomed. 'I'd rather have stayed black' is a typical response, though many negro women, particularly older ones, have often been surprised and pleased by the obvious lack of wrinkles in their newly-acquired white skin—the envy of their naturally-white friends of similar age.

It is quite clear that among both black and white peoples there is a remarkable ambivalence towards skin colour. On every holiday beach whites can be seen undergoing remarkable sufferings to acquire a dark sun tan. And many black people spend a great deal of money buying skin bleaches like those advertised in the magazine *Ebony*—'to clear away unnaturally dark areas.' In America, Africa and Asia today there are ever-increasing sales of these bleaching creams. And yet in neighbouring columns of this same magazine, there are advertisements for products for darkening the skin. At least one manufacturing chemist believes he has at last identified a truly universal demand—and has produced a pill which will provide everyone, black or white, with a neutral bronze skin—a pill, in fact, to make coffee coloured people of us all.

We noted earlier the very small skull of Erasmus. There was however another respect in which nature had been particularly unkind to him; he had a markedly unbalanced and asymmetrical face—the right half being considerably broader than the left. It is interesting to discover how very

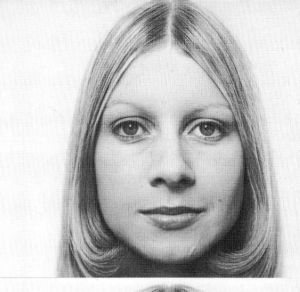

Skin and bone

Many faces are surprisingly asymmetrical and sometimes people feel that they have one side which is 'better' than the other. Many would no doubt like to reshape their faces using only their two 'good' sides. The results could be surprising

1 The natural face

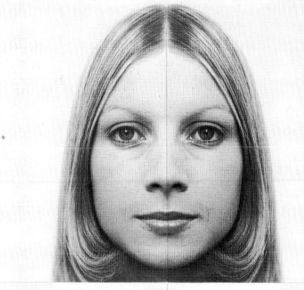

2 Composite made up of two left halves of the same face

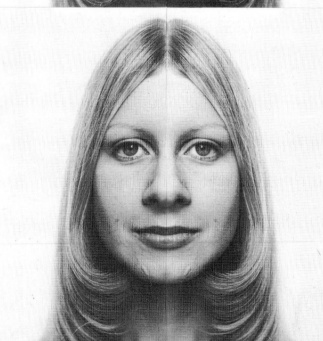

3 Composite made up of two right halves of the same face

few faces there are which are perfectly symmetrical. Indeed facial asymmetry is commonly quite marked, as our illustrations show. A face made up from two left halves (one of the left halves. having been reversed in a mirror) is often quite different from the same person's face constructed from two right halves. Wolff, who first noticed this fact, advanced the interesting, but unlikely, theory that the 'true' face, representing the conscious everyday personality, was the 'double-right'. By contrast, the 'double-left' face, he believed, was expressive of 'the darker, deeper unconscious parts of the individual's nature'.

But the essential individuality of a face depends on a great deal more than just size and symmetry. Its character is determined by the unique pattern created by its features. And it is not so much the detail of these features, nor even the individual spacing between one feature and another, so much as the *interrelationships* between all of them taken together, which enables us to recognise the face of a friend— or to recall the face of, say, a criminal. The detail is quite subordinate to the pattern; we meet very few faces in ordinary life which have such unusual single features—large noses or small eyes or bat-ears—as to make the face recognisable or memorable on the basis of these details alone. The supreme importance of this factor of 'pattern' is made clear in a striking way by our illustration of Abraham Lincoln. The electronic engineers of the Bell Telephone Laboratories who produced this 'portrait' deliberately omitted every single detailed element of the face—yet they managed to produce a 'pattern' which somehow captures the unique quality of Lincoln's face. It is the neglect of this element of 'pattern' which has rendered the 'Identikit' and 'Photofit' methods so much less useful to the police than they might otherwise have been in criminal identification, but it is not only in recognition that pattern is important. The judgements we make about people—rightly or wrongly, fairly or unfairly—are based on our sensitivity to this *total configuration* of the face, a fact which the old physiognomists completely failed to appreciate. They tried to deduce character from individual anatomical features—from a large nose, or narrow eyes or a 'weak chin'. In later chapters we shall see how, in reality, our judgements of other people—often

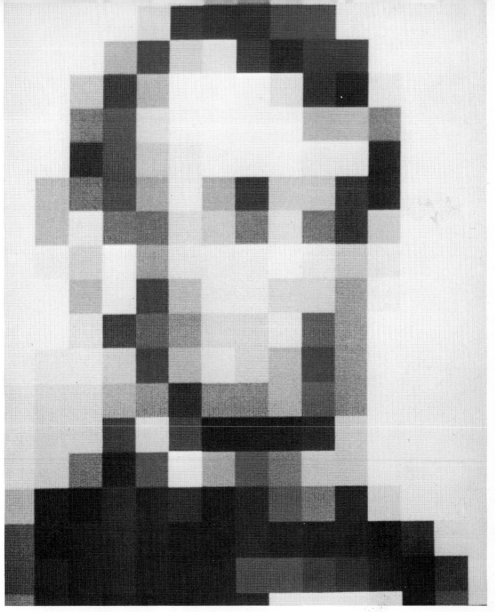

highly successful judgements—are based on a great deal more than the single individual details of skin and bone. But before we can begin to discuss this important question of the relationship between facial appearance and character, we shall need to consider much more fully the remarkable variety in facial appearance which is brought about by two quite separate, but highly important influences: on the one hand, by perfectly natural differences of sex, age and race, and on the other by man's own artificial attempts to 'improve' on nature.

2 Sex, age and race

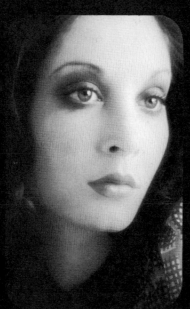

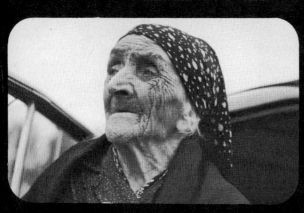

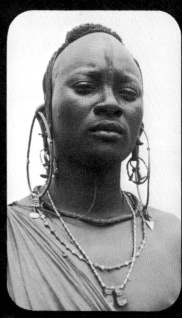

The great glory of the female face is the clarity, smoothness and fineness of its skin. Yet it has other important, though less obvious, distinctions from the face of the male. It is, for example, usually smaller in overall size—only about four fifths the size of the male. In the features, too, there are size differences; the female nose is smaller, even *proportionately* smaller than that of the male. It is also proportionately wider. Again, there are differences in the shape of the nose; the female nose is more concave and its bridge more depressed. It is interesting to reflect that these three great distinguishing characteristics of the female nose—smallness, wideness and concavity are, as we shall see, exactly those which are so pronounced in children. In an adult of either sex these characteristics are likely to contribute to an impression of both youthfulness and femininity. But there are yet other features which differ in the two sexes. The mouth is relatively smaller in females, and the upper lip often shorter. Both the jaw and the brow-ridges, too, are less pronounced. Not only is the female brow less prominent, however, it tends also to support scantier eyebrows—which often become even thinner with increasing age. By contrast, the hairs of the male brow are generally thinner in youth and tend to grow thicker, longer and coarser with age. Female eyelashes are longer and stronger than those of young males, although in later life both female eyelashes and eyebrows become thinner. There are sex differences in the eyes themselves. Female eyes are larger. The thinner, more delicate, and more transparent tissues which surround them are also much more responsive to slight changes in health and blood circulation, and so from time to time appear shaded in girls with pale skin. Though sometimes unwelcome, this occasional, natural eye-shading is a strong feminine signal. And so, in the young particularly, there are several reasons why the whole female eye region appears darker than that of the male: the stronger eyebrows and eyelashes combine with the darker irises and often dark skin surrounding the eye to create a truly distinguishing characteristic of the young female—a dark eye-zone. The widespread use of mascara and similar dark eye-cosmetics becomes very much easier to understand, as does the dangerous habit, popular in the seventeenth century, of dropping the drug belladonna into

Opposite:
A European model

Milanese centenarian.

A member of the Gogo tribe of Tanzania

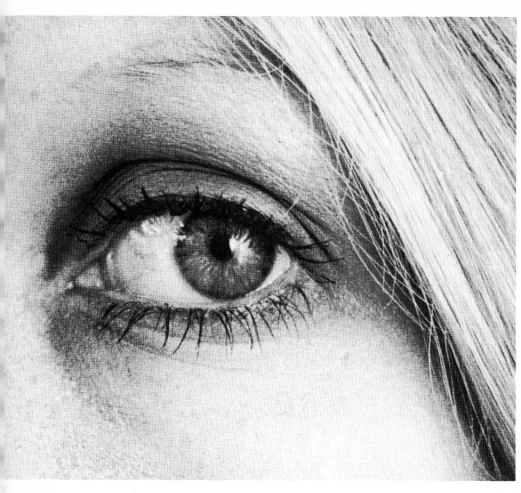

The naturally dark eye region of the young female is a strong feminine signal, an effect which may be strengthened by the judicious use of eye-cosmetics

The movements of loosely flowing hair and ear ornaments may give an illusion of stillness—and so of femininity—to the face

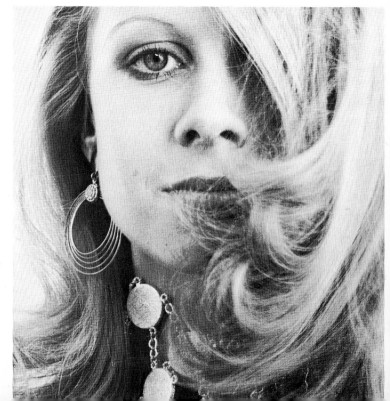

the eyes to increase their brilliance. This drug achieved its darkening effect by dilating the pupil—a dangerous process, which robbed the eye for a time of its natural reflex protection against bright light, and also, as we now know, encouraged the blinding disease of glaucoma.

The smoothness of the female face owes much to the fact that its muscles are less substantial than those of the male, and better hidden by fatty tissue. These differences have an important effect on the perception of facial movement: small muscular movements in the female face are much less obvious than similar movements in a male, and equivalent muscular movements are much less likely to produce wrinkling in the female than they are in the skinnier male. This facial movement effect is a highly important one in sexual recognition. Faces which are highly mobile, with much furrowing, are much more likely to be perceived as 'male' than are smooth, unruffled faces. Experiments by the writer have confirmed that a high degree of facial movement leads to an impression of masculinity; whilst lack of movement generally leads to quite the opposite. It follows, therefore, that cosmetics and indeed any other device which reduces apparent movement will strongly enhance the impression of femininity. Hence the popularity among women, for thousands of years, of thick paste cosmetics and mobile ear pendants—not to mention loosely flowing hair.

Some of the most interesting characteristics of the human face, however, are those produced simply by the passage of time itself. Many of the changes brought about by age, such as greying of hair and wrinkling of skin, are easy enough to see. But some of the effects of ageing are not nearly so obvious. The shape and proportions of the face, as we have noted, change a great deal between babyhood and old age. The distance from the level of the eyes to the level of the nostrils grows steadily throughout infancy—much more so, proportionally, than the rest of the face. As the baby loses his 'sucking pads' the height of the middle part of his face increases and continues to do so until well into adolescence. The shape of the baby's nose, too, is markedly different from that of the adult: it is small, wide, and nearly always concave, with a sunken bridge. In later life there is often a good deal of broadening, flattening and even wrinkling of the

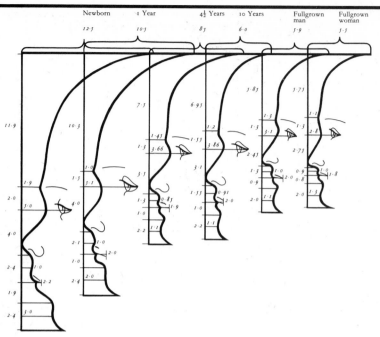

Facial proportions change a great deal between babyhood and maturity: the nose becomes proportionally much larger and the forehead proportionally smaller

nose. The eyes, also, may change considerably in old age. Their lustre diminishes—and the white sclerotic membranes, which in youth were tinged with blue, develop a tired yellow cast caused by changes in the tiny blood vessels. Changes usually occur in the coloured iris of the eyes, and the clear area in the centre of the eye, the pupil, often becomes clouded. *Around* the eyes, too, there are often marked changes, like the wrinkling of the delicate tissues of the eyelids.

The really striking changes brought about by ageing, in fact, are those which occur in the skin. The skin of the child possesses remarkable elasticity: it returns quickly to its natural contour after being displaced. In mature adults it is much more sluggish; and in old age it may take many seconds to return to its normal position after displacement. With loss of elasticity there comes also an increasing tendency for the skin to crease under the influence of the muscles, usually in the same place, forming wrinkles and coarse folds or *rugae,* which can be neither prevented nor removed, except perhaps by surgery. Unlike some of the other marks of age, such as greying hair, they defy all attempts at concealment. As the Spanish proverb has it, 'the hair deceives, the wrinkles undeceive.'

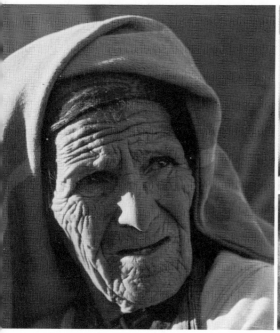

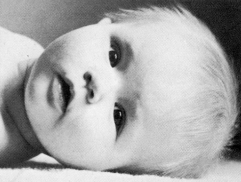

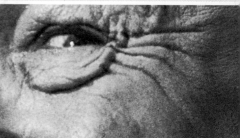

The first of the wrinkles to arrive are often the transverse lines of the forehead—which appear in most males by the age of forty—and sometimes a good deal sooner. The naso-labial furrow, from the nose to the outer corner of the lips, is often another early arrival—though, as with all facial characteristics, there are, of course, broad individual variations. The tissues around the eyes are especially susceptible to wrinkling; 'crows feet' often form at the sides—but again much depends on the individual's skin tonus and on the quality of the underlying tissue.

Some of the more subtle and interesting age-changes in the skin, however, are those which occur in its opacity and colour. The tiny capillaries and blood vessels of the skin sometimes become more and more visible with the passing of the years; the skin of the old is often paper-thin and translucent. But there is so much diversity in all the physical effects of ageing. The kind of work one does, for example, is an important factor; another is climate. Consequently the outdoor worker tends to keep his fresh, young-looking colour much longer than the sedentary worker. Chronic ill-health often leaves clear marks on the face, as does a life-time of careless diet and self-indulgence. Excess of alcohol is a well-known cause of skin changes of a more-or-less

Left An old Berber woman from Morocco

Top At six months the skin is fine and all contours full and rounded

Bottom Among the first of the wrinkles to appear are the familiar 'crow's feet'

permanent kind. But even here constitution is all-important: individuals vary a great deal in their response to physiological abuse. Many heavy drinkers retain fresh, unmarked features until the end of their days, whereas others, less fortunate, seem to light up their nose like a beacon with the mildest excess. It has often been suggested that a lifetime of dissipation and neglect leave ineradicable marks on the face. But this widely-held belief is difficult either to prove or disprove, and must, at least, be held suspect; the so-called 'marks of a careworn life' may be no more than the ordinary healthy furrows and wrinkles to which many individuals are constitutionally predisposed.

Enormous constitutional differences are to be found between individuals of similar age and racial group in both texture and wrinkling of skin and in freshness of colouring. A great variety of facial movements can readily be observed in ordinary conversation. Some people, whom we might describe as 'facialisers', move their foreheads and cheeks, and sometimes even their whole face, a great deal when expressing their feelings or emphasising a point. On the other hand, there are many people—'internalisers' they might be called—who seem automatically to restrict their facial movement; they make good poker players, but unresponsive conversationalists. It is tempting to conclude that their feelings are somehow dissipated internally—unlike the 'facialisers', whose tensions seem to be released to some degree through their facial musculature. It seems much more likely to be the combination of this 'facialising' habit with particular constitutional processes which produces the 'wrinkled face of care'. There are countless people who have lived the happiest of lives whose faces are completely smothered with characterful wrinkles. And there are countless 'internalisers' who have suffered a lifetime of poverty and despair but whose faces are still velvet-smooth in old age. As in so many aspects of human life, general vigour and constitution play a crucial part.

It is interesting to reflect on the causes of age changes in the skin. Why do the tissues sometimes change so much as age advances? Alex Comfort believes that there are three possible explanations. The first is the old suggestion, made long ago by Francis Bacon, that the body gradually loses its

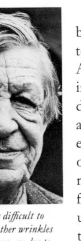

It is often difficult to judge whether wrinkles and furrows are due to age, a natural predisposition, or suffering, hardship and care

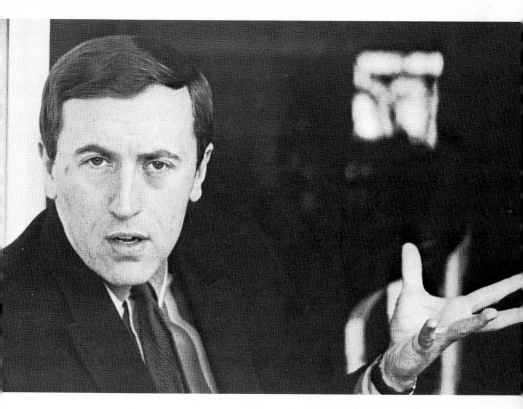

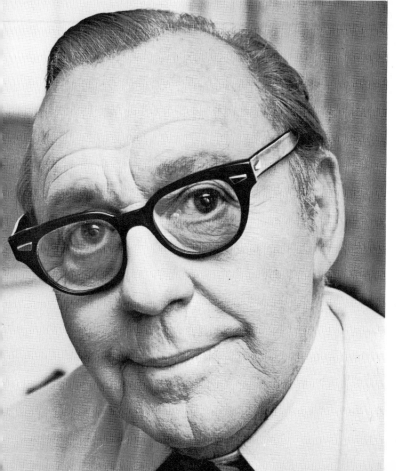

David Frost: the style
of the vigorous
'facialiser' is part of
his professional image

Jack Benny employs to
great effect the dead-pan
style of the 'internaliser'

vigour because of the dying-out of cells which, for some reason, are not replaced. It is now known that many cells of the body are of this non-multiplying, non-reproducing type. The cells of the brain, for example, are irretrievably lost in this way at the rate of tens of thousands per day. (Fortunately, we start off in life with hundreds of millions.) But whether this kind of loss accounts for the changes in the face's skinny covering is not yet known. A second, more modern, theory suggests that the skin is steadily renewed, but that the dying cells are replaced by newly-born cells which, for some reason, are never as lively and vigorous as the original cells. Some researchers have suggested that these new cells are, in fact, rather poor copies of the originals. A third theory holds that there are chemical changes in the constitution of the substances, such as collagen, which make up the tissues and the skin. Chemical changes of this kind are certainly known to occur in the blood vessels—it is these in fact which are responsible for the hardening of the arteries. But whether, and to what degree, these collagen changes are responsible for the wrinkles of old age is still not clear. It may well be that all three kinds of mechanism are at work simultaneously.

The interesting suggestion that ageing is controlled by the pituitary gland has arisen from studies of the rare disease *progeria,* in which there is grossly precocious development, premature ageing and early death. A child suffering from this condition died recently in Brazil at the age of twelve. All his secondary teeth had grown and were yellowing by the time he was six months old. His hair had turned white and was falling out before he was two years old. Before he was ten, his skin was wrinkled and dry, and his arteries were hardened like those of an old man. The pituitary gland, which is usually blamed for this condition, is known to perform many subtle and delicate functions. As well as being the chief controller of the other ductless glands of the body, it exerts an influence on yet another structure, the hypo-thalamus, which is known to be a part of the time-keeping system of the body. There is growing evidence, in fact, that different individuals do tend to live at different rates—and that 'years of age' is only a poor and rough guide to physical condition. What matters most seems to be not so much

'chronological age' as 'physiological age'. A great deal of
research effort is currently being applied to these questions,
though some authorities, including Alex Comfort, would
like to see a much greater proportion of the effort devoted
to the psychological problems of adjustment to old age and
not just to physical changes.

But the changes we can observe during ageing are much
more subtle than any discussion of mere tissue-changes
would suggest. Over the course of life there are progressive
alterations in the patterns of muscular movements used to
express feelings and to make facial communications. It is
these changing physical patterns of emotional expression
which often provide our strongest and most valuable clues
to a person's age. And what a difference there is between the
emotional expression of the mature adult and the child. The
young baby expresses his displeasure with irrepressible
intensity: there is no subtlety in his facial activity, no modu-
lation of movement by thought or reflection, no faint
movements requiring skilled decoding by the observer.
Indeed, the child is quite incapable of making fine muscular
movements. As childhood advances, however, more
subtle patterns become possible; a wider spectrum of expression becomes available. Despair, suspicion, hopefulness
and many other subtle shades of feeling can be expressed in
recognisably different ways. At the time of adolescence
strange new emotions arise, each with its own complex form
of facial expression. This is the time of life when the face can
be all too expressive—often to the severe discomfiture of
the embarrassed adolescent struggling hard to conceal his
feelings. With increasing maturity, however, a fine balance is
gradually established between sensibility and control—
between the emotions and the will. And it is often at this
time of life, in early adulthood, when the richest and most
exciting facial changes are to be seen. Even the colouring of
the face is more subtle—some artists maintain that the portraiture of the teens and twenties needs a lighter, more skilful
brush, a much more delicately varied palette. The transient
changes of expression and colour in the face before the age
of thirty are richer than any to be found thereafter. Yet these
subtle patterns of youth submit, all too soon, to two kinds
of attack which act in parallel. The first stems from the

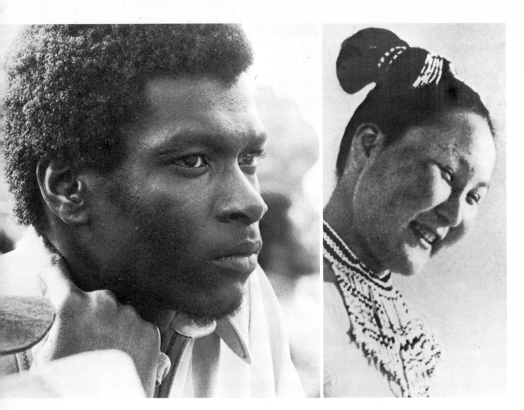

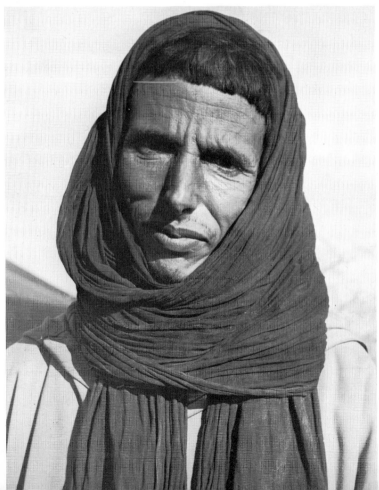

Top left *Negroid peoples often but not always have a broad nose with wide depressed root and broad concave bridge*

Top right *Many Mongoloid peoples have a broad head and a deeply-sunken nose*

Right *A Regibat tribesman from Southern Morocco*

reason and the will: considered judgement restrains the display of private feelings—experience soon teaches the advantages of the 'poker face'. The second follows upon structural changes; thickening of tissues, increasing flaccidity of muscles and loss of elasticity in the skin mean that gross movements must now supplant subtle ones. Where once a slight but complex change of expression would suffice to convey a message, stronger movements are now needed, not only of the face, but of the whole head, perhaps even of the limbs. Old people have a much-diminished repertoire of facial expressions; they need to make their point over and over again, intensifying their message by dull repetition. Expression in the aged seems almost to have come full-circle; it has returned to the intensity and poverty of that of the young child.

Of all the differences which occur in the human face those due to race are by far the most obvious and the most impressive. But race is extremely difficult to define and its nature and origins have been the subject of much controversy. In the Bible it is written that all mankind is descended from the three sons of Noah: Ham, Shem and Japhet—whose descendants produced the three races of mankind, the Hamitics, the Semitics and the Japhetics. The Hamitics included the Berbers of North Africa, the Egyptians and the Somali. The Semitic group included the Arabian, Abyssinian and Hebrew peoples. The Japhetics were the Celts, the Teutons, the Slavs, the Italians, and the peoples of Iran. Although scholars in the past have sometimes found these classifications useful there has been much controversy and disagreement about the true nature of race, and few scientists today are prepared to accept the Biblical division. It is surprising to discover just how many different criteria have been proposed at one time or another for classifying the peoples of the world into races. In the eighteenth century, the botanist Linnaeus was impressed by the large variations which he found in *skin colour* in different lands and made the proposal that we should classify people into 'black-skinned', 'white-skinned' and 'yellow-skinned'.

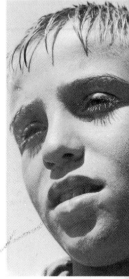

A boy of Caucasoid type from Myconos

Modern students of race, however, pay much more attention to questions of shape and proportion of the head and face. Measurements have shown, for example, that

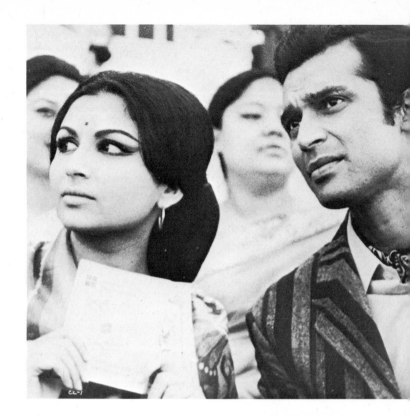

Two young faces of modern India from the film Company Limited

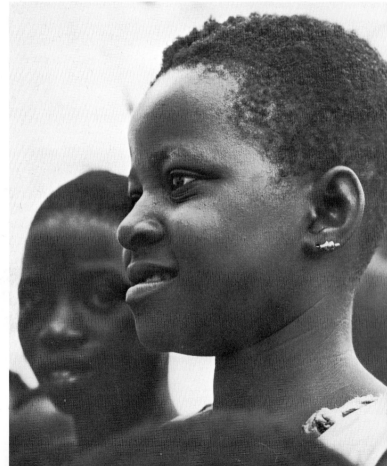

Right:
African boy

Opposite *An American Plains Indian of the 19th century*

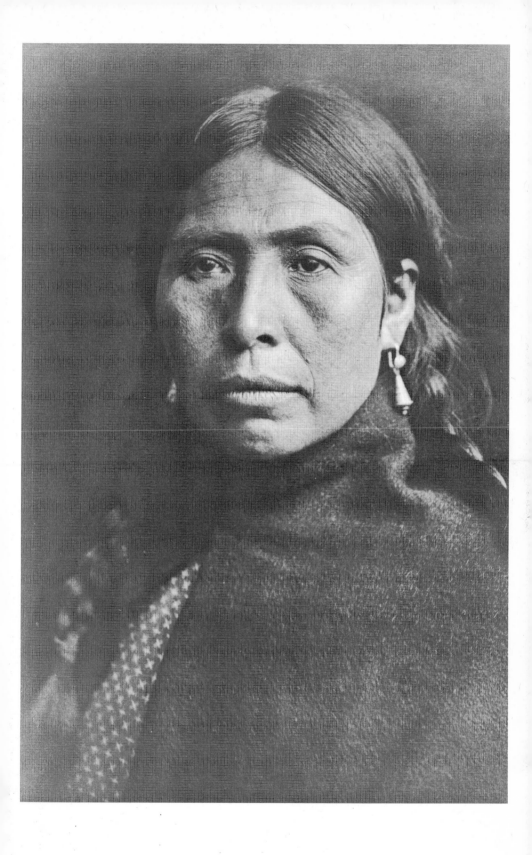

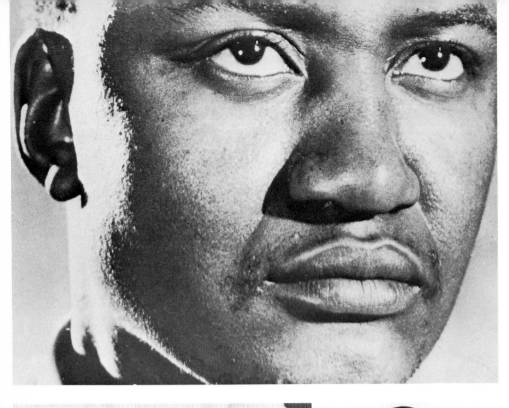

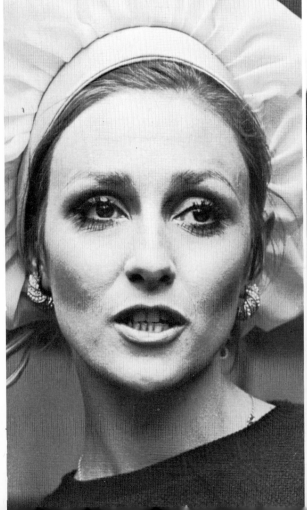

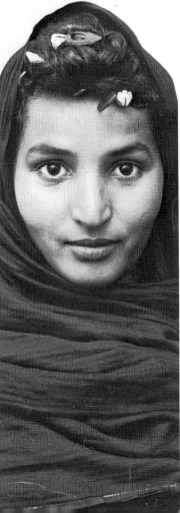

Europeans and Negroes often tend to have long heads, whereas many Chinese have relatively broad heads. Both the length and breadth of the face, however, vary considerably even within single racial sub-groups. Herodotus discovered considerable variations in the thickness of the skulls he examined. He observed that the ancient Egyptians had thick skulls and the Persians thin: this, he believed, was because they belonged to different races. Others have been interested not so much in the skull or in the general size and shape of the head as a whole as in its *individual features*. The French anthropologist Topinard, for example, became interested in the rich variety of shapes to be found in human *noses*. He was the first to make detailed studies of nasal forms and had much to say on the relative beauty of each. He developed a comprehensive scheme for classifying nasal shapes, and anthropologists have since found his system a useful one. Nowadays, like Topinard, they distinguish narrow nosed or 'leptorrhine' people (such as white Caucasians) from broad nosed or 'platyrrhine' people (such as Negroids). Between these two types are the medium nosed or 'meso-rrhine' peoples (such as the Mongoloid peoples of Central Asia). The narrow-nosed Caucasians often have a high nasal root and high bridge, and frequently, too, a long tip to the nose. Negroid peoples, by contrast, often have a broad nose with a wide, depressed root, a broad, concave bridge, and a thick tip. The Mongoloids generally have a nose which is quite concave and often deeply sunken in the face. The bridge is low and narrow, the wings of the nose are thin, and the tip is often small. The leptorrhines are usually defined as being 'those with a nasal index below 70' (the nasal index is calculated by dividing the width of the nose by its length and multiplying by 100); the mesorrhines are those between 70 and 84; and the platyrrhines those above 84. Many intermediate and 'mixed nasal types' have also been described: European 'Alpines', for example, have a high nasal index, a straight profile to the nose, and a thick tip. American Plains Indians have a convex bridge, a long, downward-pointing tip and large wings to the nostrils, which flare considerably. But there are infinite variations.

Many ethnologists believe that variations in the *hair*, too, provide a useful basis for racial classification. Hair certainly

Opposite:
Top *South African Negro from the film* Let My People Go

Bottom left *A European model, of typical Caucasian type*

Bottom right *A Mauritanian woman*

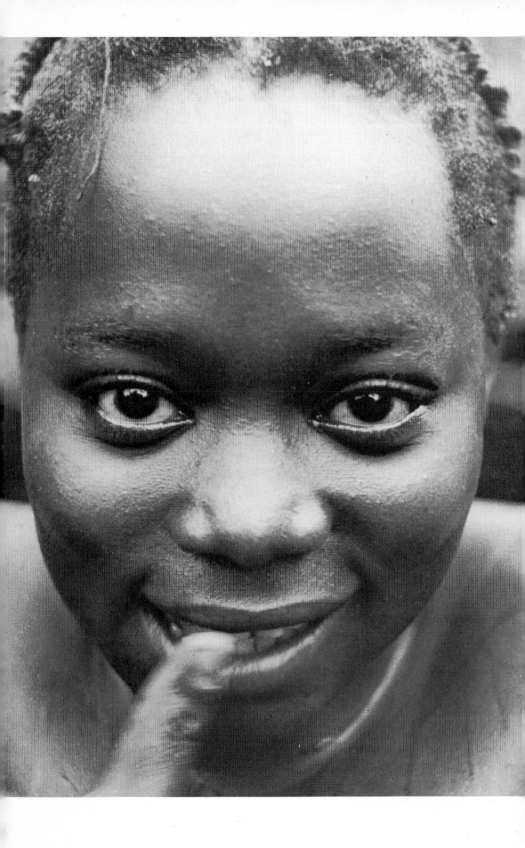

varies widely among the different peoples of the world. The French ethnographer Deniker described what he believed to be the six 'major types' of hair and no less than seventeen 'minor' categories. He differentiated hair which was straight and smooth (such as is often found in China) from hair which was wavy (as in Western Europe), curly (as in Western Europe), woolly (as in Africa), or frizzy (as in some other parts of Africa). The cross-section of individual hairs also showed interesting variations; negroid hairs tending to be flat in cross-section whereas caucasoid hair was round in section.

Eye-colour, again, has been much studied in relation to race. It has been found, in general, to follow hair colour—pale eyes occurring with pale hair and dark eyes with darker hair—though there are many exceptions to the rule, as indeed there are to most generalisations about race. There are, for example, many pale eyes to be found among the dark-haired people of Brittany and Cornwall. But one of the most remarkable discoveries about eye pigmentation has been that all the many subtle and varied shades of eye colour which exist are produced by just one single brown pigment: melanin. Turquoise-blue, green, grey, hazel and dark brown are all brought about simply by differences in the *quantity* of melanin present in the iris. In the deep brown eyes of the Negro the melanin is richly supplied. It is distributed throughout the whole iris—not only in the outer and the middle layers but also in the deeper parts—providing Negro peoples with ample protection against the harsh tropical sun. In lighter-eyed peoples from cloudier latitudes the melanin is missing from the outermost layer—and in blue-eyed peoples the melanin pigment is to be found only in the inner layers of the iris. This sparseness of pigment in blue-eyed peoples contributes to the difficulty they sometimes have in seeing clearly and focusing their eyes in bright sunshine—and gives them a special need for protective sunglasses.

There are some interesting racial variations to be found in the tissues around the eyes. One interesting example is the fold of skin which commonly appears slantwise across the outside of the eye in Eastern Asiatic peoples. This is the so-called 'epicanthic fold', which exerts a powerful effect on

Opposite *The dark eyes of this girl from the Cameroons are deeply pigmented with melanin to protect them from the intense equatorial sun* facial appearance. It is often a striking feature in Chinese and Japanese faces. But there are racial differences in other features too. Even lips show remarkable racial variations. Full and thick lips are to be found among the Negroes of Africa, whereas thin, pale 'Simian' lips are much more frequently found among Europeans. Ears also vary considerably in size and shape—largest among the yellow-brown Asiatic peoples, and smallest in the Negroids, who sometimes have little or no lobe at all.

Many feature-differences such as these have been proposed at one time or another as a basis for classifying mankind into 'races'. But it is quite clear by now that any attempt to use a single feature as a criterion of race is doomed to failure. Modern ethnologists have reached the conclusion that nothing less than the collection or the *pattern* of characteristics can be relied upon to provide any indication of racial membership.

Still there has been such confusion, even in recent years, about the true nature of race that the United Nations actually appointed an international group of experts in anthropology, ethnology and the social sciences to provide a definitive statement. The result, the UNESCO *Statement on Race,* was published in 1950. The scientists expressed their concern in this about some of the highly undesirable and misinformed ideas about race which were still current—ideas indeed which, as the report said, should be regarded as little more than 'myth':

> The myth of race has created an enormous amount of human and social damage. In recent years it has taken a heavy toll in human lives and caused untold suffering. It still prevents the normal development of millions of human beings and deprives civilization of the effective cooperation of productive minds.

The statement made it clear that the term 'race' is commonly used quite incorrectly:

> Unfortunately . . . to most people, a race is any group of people whom they choose to describe as a race. Thus, many national, religious, geographic, linguistic or cultural groups have, in such loose usage, been called a 'race', when obviously Americans are not a race, nor are Englishmen, nor Frenchmen, nor any other national

group. Catholics, Protestants, Moslems, and Jews are not races, nor are groups who speak English or any other language thereby definable as a race, people who live in Iceland or England or India are not races: nor are people who are culturally Turkish or Chinese, or the like thereby describable as races.

The conclusion was that the whole of mankind belongs to one single species, *homo sapiens*. This must be the case, because all members of mankind, from whatever country, can interbreed with one another. And 'there is no evidence that race mixture as such produces bad results from a biological point of view'.

So far, however, the report continues, interbreeding has tended to occur only on a limited scale, because of purely physical obstacles such as mountains and oceans. Consequently a few very large groups have tended to develop and evolve separately—and to adapt differently to the varied climatic and other conditions of their distinct continents. Not surprisingly, therefore, each of these large groups has developed certain superficial physical differences: tropical peoples, for example, have developed dark skins to protect them from the sun. Now, interesting as these differences are—and ethnologists have spent a great deal of time and energy studying and describing them—they are, as the UNESCO report makes quite clear, only superficial. They are not important. They confer no superiority or inferiority on any particular group—except in the sense that some groups have made a superior adaptation to local conditions: Negroes, for example, are much better able to stand strong sunlight and Eskimos much better able to withstand cold. It would be better, the UNESCO report concludes, if we were to think of race in these geographical terms. Indeed, it would be preferable 'when speaking of human races to drop the term "race" altogether, and speak of "ethnic groups".'

Physical differences apart, therefore, the interesting question now arises as to whether there are any important corresponding psychological and temperamental differences. On this issue, the UNESCO report is quite clear:

As for personality and character these may be considered raceless. In every human group a rich variety of character

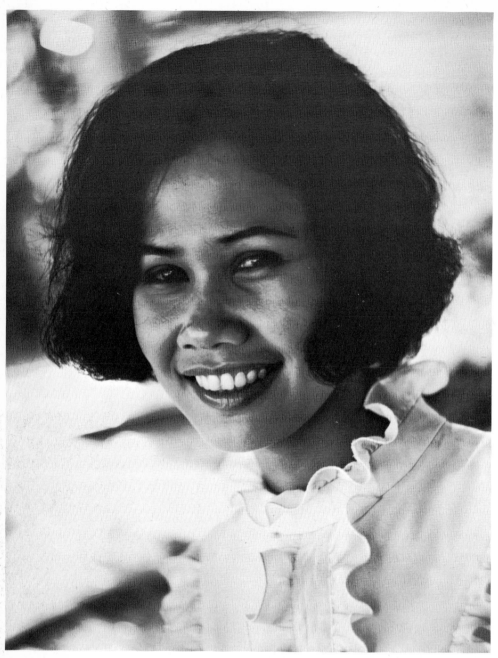

types will be found, and there is no reason for believing that any human group is richer than any other in these respects.

Yet many people do believe that such temperamental differences exist. It has often been suggested, in discussions about Europeans, for example, that dark-haired Italians and

Spaniards are from birth more talkative, sociable and vivacious, excitable and impetuous than fair-haired, long-headed, long-faced Northern Europeans, who are often expected to be much quieter and more introverted, given more to reflection than to active social discussion. As the UNESCO report explains, however, groups of people like these have been kept together by such geographical circumstances as mountains and oceans, and subjected to common climate, common habitat and common environmental influences. It is hardly surprising, therefore, that individuals within each group should have acquired, during their lifetime, characteristics favoured and encouraged by their own particular environment. It would be very reasonable to expect every Italian, for example, to become more talkative and more sociable simply because he lives in conditions where sociability and gregariousness are encouraged by ease of social contact in a warm and friendly climate. But group characteristics of this kind are, at root, *environmental*. They are not due to inborn physical factors associated with race. Furthermore we must beware of expecting every Italian we meet to be talkative, or every Eskimo to be silent. Individual differences within every group of people are truly enormous; for example, every Italian is different from his fellows. The detailed history of every man's own personal life needs to be considered. As well as having been under the influence of the general ethnic 'external environment' which bears upon everyone in his group, every man gradually constructs his own 'personal environment', made up of his experiences, successes, failures, ideas, ideals, worries and preoccupations, which, as we shall see in a later chapter, may very well be reflected in his personality and possibly even in his facial appearance. The UNESCO report makes it quite clear that the mere fact of a man's belonging to a particular ethnic group and possessing the corresponding physical features tells us nothing whatsoever about his character and temperament. Race and temperament are unrelated; all kinds of temperament can be found in every race. As the UNESCO report declared, 'the scientific investigations of recent years fully support the dictum of Confucius . . . "Men's natures are alike; it is their habits that carry them far apart."'

Opposite:
A high proportion of faces incorporate more than one so-called racial characteristic. The face of this attractive girl photographed in Thailand contains 'Caucasoid' and 'Negroid' as well as 'Mongoloid' characteristics

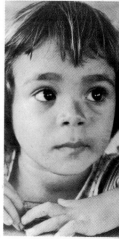

Nationality, like racial origins, is often quite undetectable: a young schoolgirl from Brazil

3 Primitive elaboration

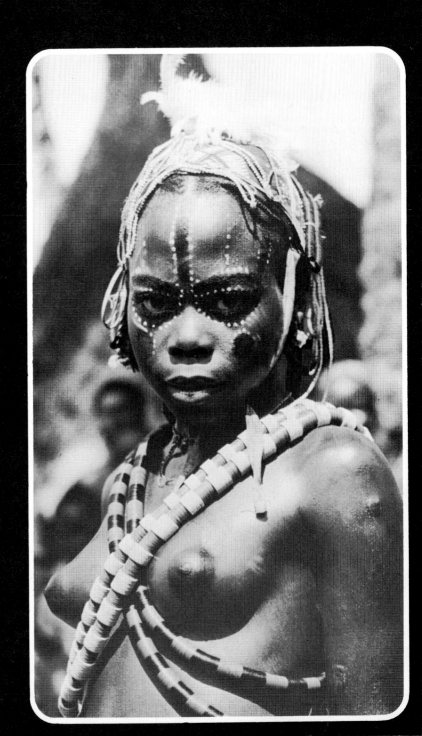

The desire to alter the face is universal; in every country and in every age examples of facial elaboration can be found. Often the objective is to acquire greater beauty in the eyes of one's companions—though, as we shall see, this is by no means the only motive. Yet even the pursuit of beauty leads to an incredible variety of facial embellishments; and conceptions of beauty are unbelievably varied, even within a single society. As the Scottish philosopher David Hume recognised more than two hundred years ago, there are no universally acceptable standards. Beautiful faces are simply those which satisfy taste, and taste, in the words of the anthropologist Sumner, 'is not an independent reality but is relative, local and highly personal. Standards of beauty differ widely and have little in common; they may be opposite and contradictory.' So impressed in fact was Darwin by the regional and continental differences which he found in ideals of beauty that he was even led to conclude that the separation of mankind into disparate races had actually been brought about by these widely varying local standards. Some strange reasons are sometimes offered by people themselves to explain their preferences. One example is given by Letourneau:

> The Kirghiz think that their race, the Mongolian, offers the most finished type of human beauty, because the bony structure of their face resembles that of a horse—the greatest masterpiece of all creation.

Australian natives laugh at the sharp noses of Europeans because they are 'tomahawk noses'. They deliberately flatten their own babies' noses by pressing them with the hand or by laying them flat on their faces. As Sumner has shown, primitive peoples will not hesitate to use violent means if necessary, to achieve their local ideal. They are 'quite ready to cut off all variations from it.' Some of the methods employed are, as we shall see, unbelievably cruel; even infanticide has been practised to preserve the purity and perfection of the esteemed local type.

The softness of young babies' skulls has encouraged, in many countries, the almost unbelievable custom of *deformation* of the face and head. This has usually been practised on girls to achieve beauty in the eyes of the tribe or to secure magical protection against disease. The most common

Opposite *The desire to alter the face is universal*

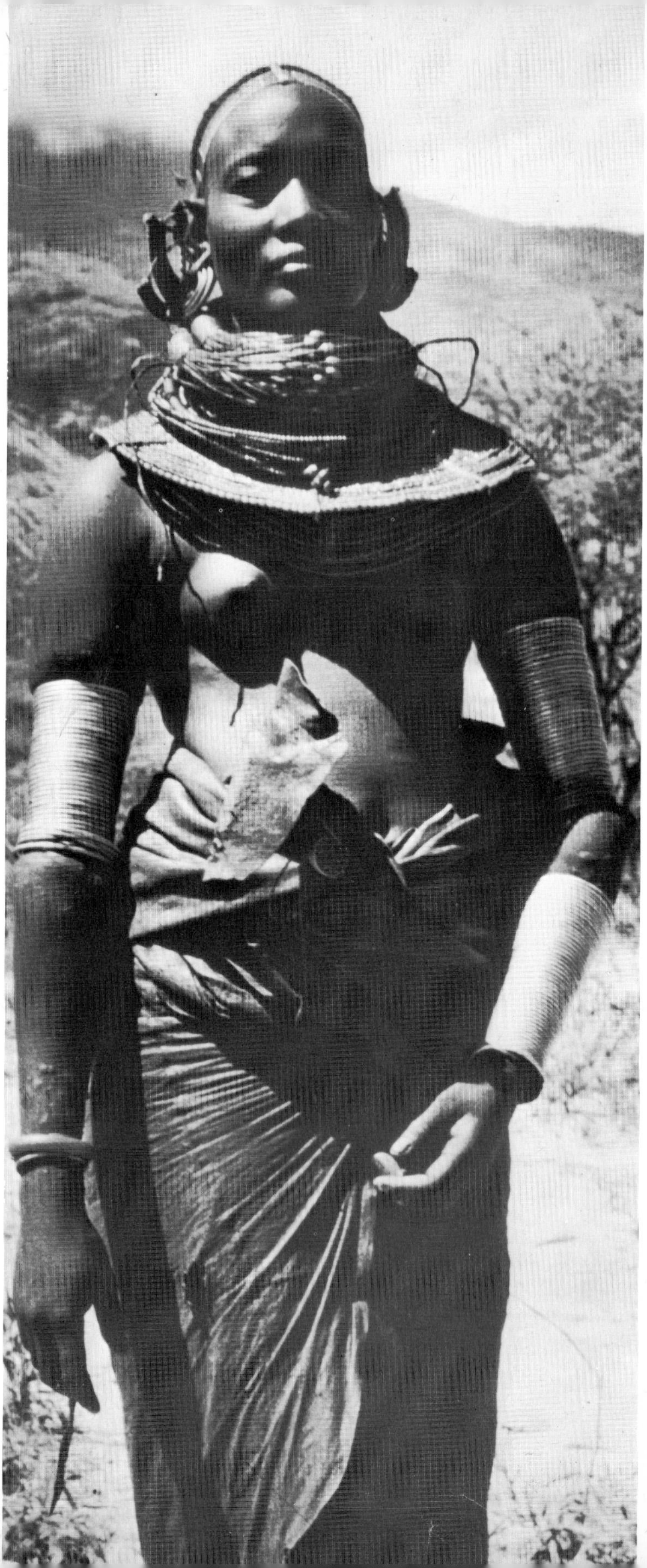

A prostitute of the Samburu tribe wearing little more than jewellery around her head and face

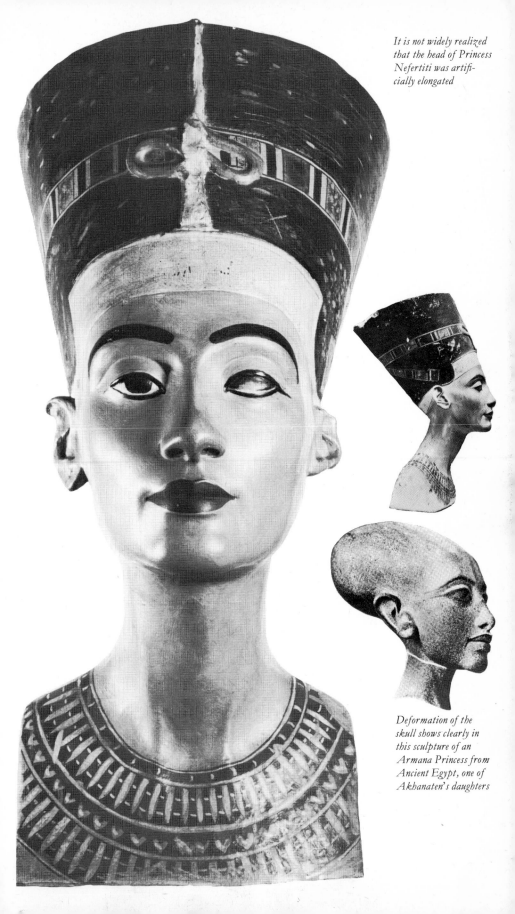

It is not widely realized that the head of Princess Nefertiti was artificially elongated

Deformation of the skull shows clearly in this sculpture of an Armana Princess from Ancient Egypt, one of Akhanaten's daughters

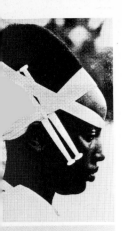

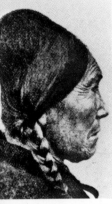

method was to apply pressure to the soft skull during the first weeks of life to make the head round, flat or elongated, according to local taste. The child was laid on its back, and the head surrounded with three flat stones; one was placed close to the crown of the head and one on either side. The forehead was then pressed with the hand and flattened. The nose, too, was carefully flattened. Head deformation is of great antiquity; it is known to have been practised in pre-neolithic Jericho. Hippocrates and Pliny both referred to the popularity of head deformation in high-born Greek and Roman families. The skull of the celebrated Egyptian princess Nefertiti was artificially deformed in this way, as also were those of the daughters of Amenhotep IV. It can still be seen among some African peoples, and in Greenland and Peru. According to Backman, it could also be seen, until quite recently, in Brittany, Normandy, and the region around Toulouse. The technique in France was to use a very tight cap secured by strings. The American Indians used a rather different method with boards secured by tapes. It is remarkable that it was possible to make such profound changes in the shape of the skull without, it seems, producing any serious damage to the brain, although epilepsy and protrusion of the eyes were sometimes the result of serious deformation.

Countless examples can be found of painful elaborations of the face. All peoples, sophisticated as well as primitive, seem prepared to go through almost unbelievable suffering in pursuit of the purely local ideals of their particular society. Beauty must be pursued at whatever price, because it confers on its possessor profound social influence, power and respect. At one time, the young Botocudo girls of Brazil willingly accepted the insertion of larger and larger discs into their lower lips until a grotesque 'spoon-bill' was produced. Among African peoples labrets such as these were even worn in pairs, which rattled together as they tried to speak. Livingstone observed that the circumference of the distorted lips might be as much as twenty-nine inches:

> The women seen at a distance and in profile seemed to be holding two saucers between their teeth. Eating was very difficult, and the woman was, to all practical intents, dumb. The labret was grossly uncomfortable; yet it was a

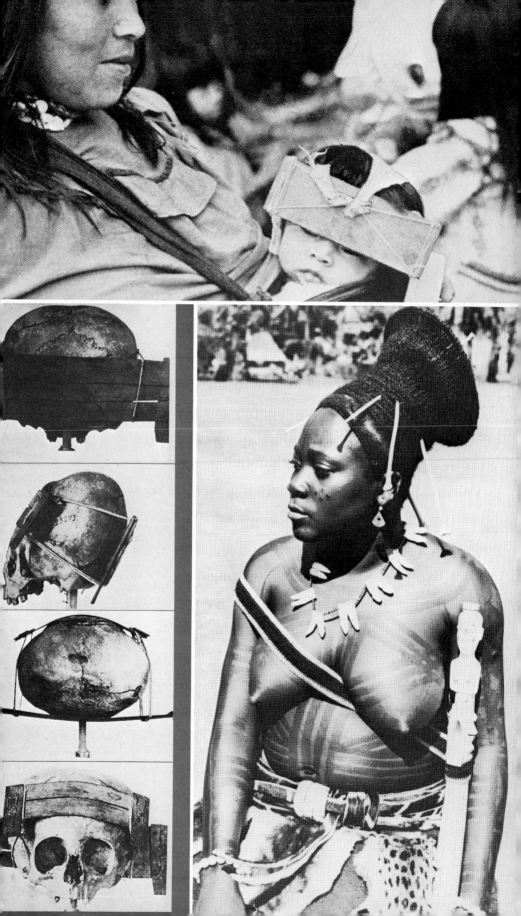

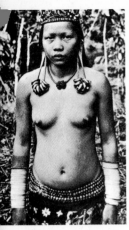

mark of honour and people who so regarded it hesitated at nothing to get it and to celebrate its attainment lavishly.

Among the Thlinkits of North-West Canada, too, the custom of wearing bone or silver labrets was once widespread. These labrets varied in size according to the rank of the wearer. Their size was increased as the woman grew older, and so it was possible to judge her age from the size of the labret she wore. Painful piercing of the nose, lips, ears and sometimes even the cheeks was once common in many countries. Considerable mutilations were undertaken without any help whatsoever from anaesthetics. Captain Cook reported that New Zealanders had enormous holes 'the diameter of a man's finger' pierced in the lobes of their ears, through which they threaded bones, coloured cloth, twigs and feathers. One man seen by Cook wore a large feather through his nose. In New South Wales, such nose ornaments were particularly common among the menfolk, though more often they consisted of bones rather than feathers. The Eskimos, like the Papuans on the other side of the world, used to thrust a sharp stick through the septum of their nose. In South America, the Cobeus, the fiercest of the Amazon tribes, made holes in their ears large enough to hold a small bunch of arrows. And in the South Pacific, as Sumner records, ear-perforation was equally common:

Into the perforations of the ears feathers, knives, rings of great weight and even casual articles, such as half-smoked cigars were inserted. A Melanesian woman was seen with a little dog hung to her ear, one of his feet being attached to the lobe. Ear-lobes were so distended that great care had to be taken in running races and other activities lest they get caught and rent asunder.

Even the eyeballs were not immune from decorative interference, as Doughty observed in 1876 among North African tribesmen:

Both men and women townsfolk and Bedouins, where they may come by it, paint the whites of their eyes blue, with kohl or antimony: thus Mohammed Ibn Rashid has his birdlike eyes painted. Not only would they be more love-looking in the eyes of the women, but they hold that this sharpens too, and will preserve, their vision.

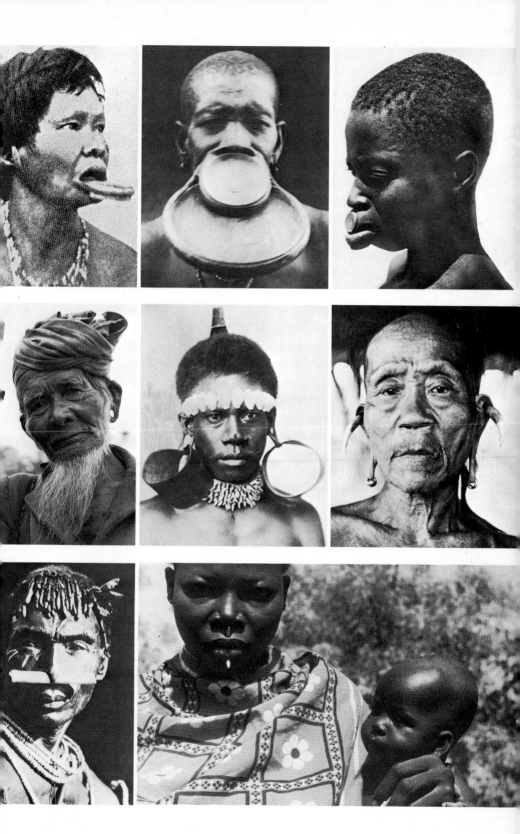

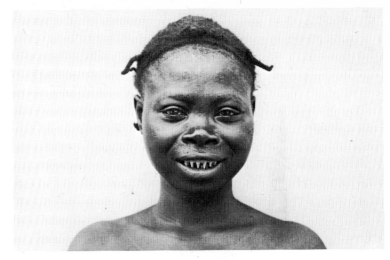

Teeth-filing: one of the more painful methods of facial elaboration

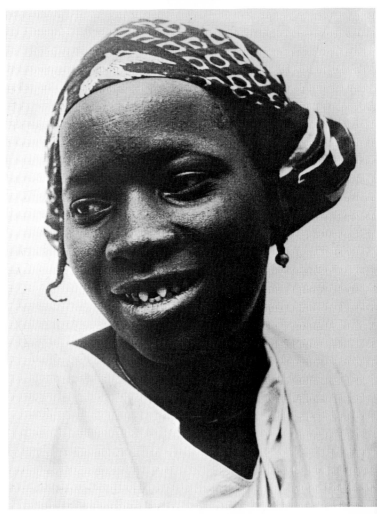

These painful facial elaborations were not always under-taken entirely in the pursuit of beauty; sometimes they had deep ritual significance. They were often an intrinsic part of initiation rites in which young people were welcomed to the privileges of adulthood. Some of the procedures used seem to us frighteningly barbaric—and yet they were cheerfully, even eagerly, endured. The native peoples of Australia and New Guinea used to celebrate the achievement of their adulthood and maturity by having their two top front teeth knocked out. And in South Africa at one time this custom was so widespread that a person who still had all his teeth was considered ugly—and would be the target for all kinds of insults. Furness described 'an ineffably excrutiating mandate of fashion' which used to be observed in Borneo:

The Ibans, not content with blackening the teeth, actually drill holes through and through the faces of the six front teeth, and therein insert plugs of brass, whereof the outer end is elaborated into stars. They then finish up by filing the teeth to sharp points! No dentist's chair can hold a more hideous torture than this. The drill—usually no more delicate an instrument than the rounded end of a file—bores directly through the sensitive pulp of the tooth, tearing and twisting a nerve so exquisitely sensitive that but to touch it starts the perspiration and seems the limit of human endurance: yet an Iban will lie serene and unquivering on the floor while his beauty is thus en-hanced by some kind and tender-hearted friend.

Another description, by Wilken, tells how, in the East Indies, the teeth were even filed off down to the gums as part of the ceremonial of wedding, puberty or mourning. He believed this filing to be a kind of self-sacrifice, like hair-offering. A tooth might sometimes be demanded, too, by a warrior as a sign of subjection. Archaeologists have found clear evidence that as long ago as 2000 BC canine teeth and incisors were being knocked out or filed down during religious ceremonies in Japan. An important motive under-ying facial disfigurements of this kind is often self-dedica-ion to a deity. Scarifications and other cruel forms of sacri-ice and self-torture are mentioned in the Bible: there are several references, for example, to 'cutting for the dead'. And in many religions facial and bodily mutilations have

been taken as showing that a proper relationship has been
established with the gods and the spirits.

One of the most popular of all methods of facial alteration, in fact, has been scarification—particularly among
peoples of dark skin, for whom it is especially attractive
because the scars reveal brightly-coloured flesh beneath.
Again, unbelievably brutal methods have been used for
cutting patterns on the face. One involved the use of a fragment of skull to produce deep wounds into which black
paint or wood ashes were then introduced. Sometimes
repeated cutting and scratching of the same scars was undertaken, leading to the formation of raised 'hypertrophic' scar
tissue. This technique was strikingly effective among
Negroid peoples, whose fibroplastic tissues especially
favour the process. In Central Africa, 'cicatrisation' such as
this was once widely used to indicate tribal affiliation or
passage through initiation rites, or even to commemorate
an important event. The Abipone people of South America
used sharp thorns and a mixture of blood and ashes to
produce their distinctive clan marks in the delicate skin of
their faces, breasts and arms. These markings were eagerly
acquired: they were valued proclamations of clan membership and proud proofs of passage through initiation rites.
Boys and girls would, later in life, enlarge their cicatrices;
any person who wished to be considered fashionable had to
work away at his scars every week or so, cutting them
deeper and putting wads into the cuts to cause the flesh to
stand up. It is interesting to note that various forms of
scarification and disfigurement have sometimes been highly
valued in Western Society: a man with a strong but damaged
face might sometimes be judged more attractive than one
with unmarked features. Lord Arlington, for example, was
once described by de Grammont thus:

> He had a scar across his nose, which was covered by a
> long patch or rather by a small plaster in form of a
> lozenge. Scars on the face commonly give a man a fierce
> and martial air, which sets him off to advantage.

Such facial markings have often brought especial esteem if
they have been acquired in honourable combat—as they are
sometimes even today by the Afghans in their festivals in
which the 'Buzkashi' game is played with murderous horse-

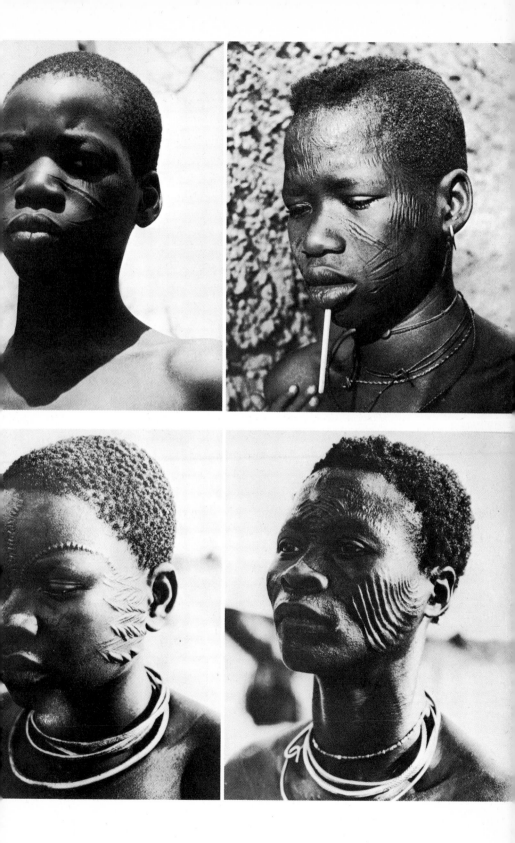

whips. Similarly, sword-scars acquired during honourable duelling were much prized by students in pre-war Germany

Of all the methods of facial decoration, however, tattooing is the most common, especially among peoples with pale skin. As Darwin observed, 'Not one great country can be named, from the Polar regions in the north to New Zealand in the south, in which the aborigines do not tattoo themselves.' Facial tattooing is of great antiquity. It was practised by the ancient Thracians, by the ancient Assyrians and by Ancient Britons. Tattoo markings can be clearly seen on ancient Egyptian paintings and monuments and on Japanese pottery made more than three thousand years ago Among the Maoris of New Zealand tattooing eventually developed into a highly advanced art form, though Polynesia and Micronesia are the classic regions for the tattoo indeed, the word 'tattoo' comes from that part of the world

The motives underlying tattooing are not hard to find there is in everyone a strong social need to be recognised received and accepted by one's group. Badges which proclaim group affiliation are, in consequence, proudly worn Sumner discovered that in Samoa a young man was, at one time, considered to be in his minority until he was tattooed he could not even think of marriage, and was constantly exposed to taunt and ridicule as being poor, low-born and 'having no rights to speak in the society of men.' When youth reached the age of sixteen, he and his friends were as anxious that he should be tattooed as soon as possible Tattoo markings sometimes served to indicate the class or clan of the wearer. Like the tragic caste-marks of India which for centuries have separated the wretched from the even-more wretched, they identified the wearer as a member of a particular sector of society. Tattoo marks might also have a very practical recognition value: special marks on particular parts of the face have been commonly used as marks of identification. The womenfolk of some African tribes used tattoo marks as a form of 'insurance'; they had a small round spot tattooed on their forehead, by which, in case of capture in tribal warfare, they would be recognised and, with luck, offered for ransom. Such marks, too, would ensure that they were not mistakenly killed in battle by their own tribesmen. In the Congo tattooing of children was regularly undertaken at a very young age so that they would not be lost among other tribes in the forest.

Facial markings have often been used to identify people with their particular totem. These were frequently the same markings as those used on canoes, totem posts, weapons and utensils and indeed many other forms of property, even wives. A man's tattoos might sometimes be used to proclaim his wealth: a poor man could afford only a few straight, coarse marks, whereas a rich man could display an impressive array of fine expensive lines. Rank and family-connections might also be recognisable from the character of the designs, and in this sense the designs were often heraldic. Restriction of tattooing to those of high social rank was sometimes rigidly enforced. One visitor to Raiatea in the nineteenth century reported that he had seen 'a native woman of naturally agreeable features, disfigured by an extensive patch of charcoal on her cheek—a punishment inflicted on her for having slightly tattooed herself, a practice forbidden in one of her lowly rank.' In some societies tattoos might record some important social feast attended. Occasionally, lines were tattooed on the face to record achievements of various kinds—such as the number of whales killed or even the number of human heads taken. Twenty-nine such lines were seen by one traveller in Indonesia and there was one old Melanesian Chief who boasted ninety-five.

But the meanings attached to facial markings are purely local. In some societies, for example, tattoo marks have been used to record *lack* of achievement—or even disgrace. One island chief who ran away from a fight was deposed and branded with two square tattoos on his face. Sometimes tattoo marks have been used for marking slaves, and in Nicaragua such tattoos were made on the face. Some of these slave marks were in the form of a cross. Yet another use for tattoo marks was as a 'signature'. One old account reported that, 'Some missionaries once bought a certain piece of land from a chief, and the tattoo marks upon the face of the seller of the land were copied on to the deed of sale, serving thereby as his signature to the contract.'

Much tattooing, however, was purely ornamental; colours were often chosen with considerable aesthetic sensitivity. Sometimes decoration was undertaken for sexual reasons. Tattooing of this kind, usually of the lips and tongue, can still be found in several parts of the world. Such decoration of the mouth region sometimes seems to carry intense sexual significance as, for example, among the Boloki, who believe that tattoos worn by men exert a powerful attraction on women. Tattoos are by no means restricted to males, of course; examples can be found where the women are tattooed and the men are not. And among some peoples a woman not tattooed as 'marriageable' might have no attraction whatsoever in the eyes of young men. On the other hand, a 'correctly' tattooed or scarified woman was the first to be wanted; it was she who brought the largest price. Special markings were sometimes made on the face at the time of marriage. In the case of girls who received unexpected and desirable offers of marriage and who could not take the usual time to acquire the necessary extensive and elaborate decorations, the operation was often driven through with relentless vigour amounting almost to torture. Girls were overpowered by female relations and forced to submit, the fevered face being dipped frequently into sea-water. As Sumner explained,

> The instant that the poor wretch of a girl was released from the hands and toes of her tormentors, she ran with the swiftness of agony to the river, there to soothe with the cool flowing water the frightful, burning ache. The absorption of so much foreign matter by the lymphatics often induced high fever; suppuration also not infrequently resulted from the septic manner in which the operation was performed; this naturally injured the sharpness of the lines. After one session, the tattooing was not resumed until the skin was entirely healed, unless an approaching marriage necessitated the utmost speed; should a woman have a child before her tattooing was completed, she was lastingly disgraced.

A sad use for tattooing was once prevalent in Australia: a woman tattooed her face to indicate that she had lost a child. But then at least perhaps her fertility was in no doubt. In several societies tattoo marks have been used to record the number of children a woman has borne.

Tattoo marks have often been believed to have had

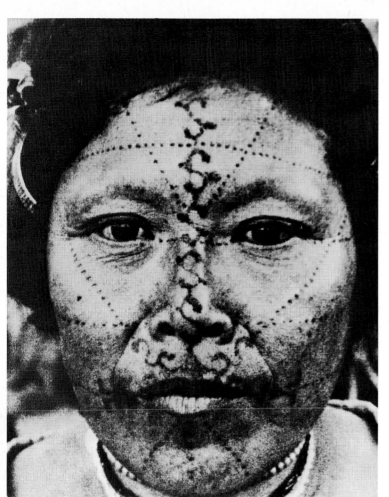

Primitive elaboration

Tattooed, geometrical pattern from South America

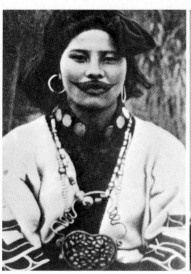

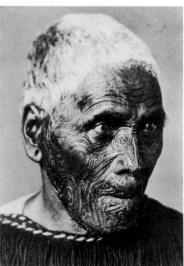

Left *Deliberate exaggeration of the mouth was once fashionable among the Ainu women of Japan. The painful tattooing process was begun by mothers when their daughters were only two years old, and often took as long as two years to complete*

Right *Among the Maoris of New Zealand, elaborate patterns such as these were considered a mark of male valour and distinction*

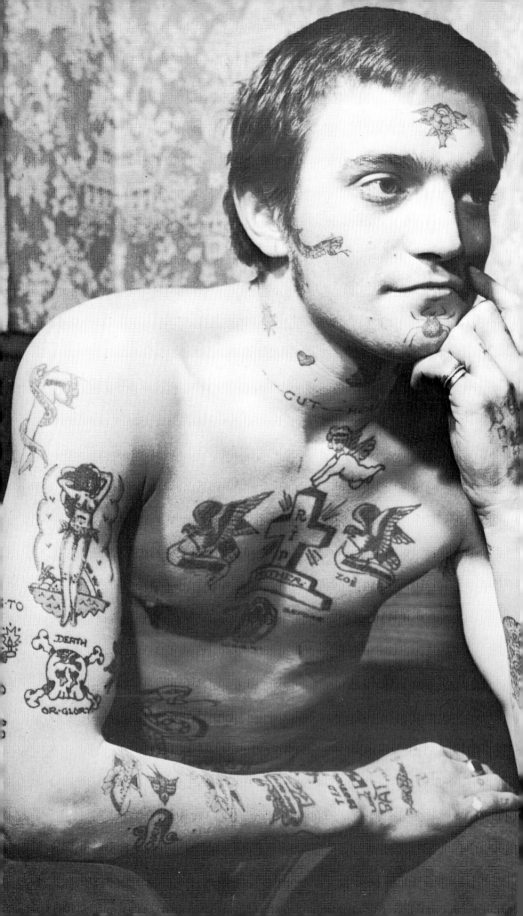

magical powers. The patterns employed had symbolic value—a bull, for example, giving the wearer virility and a scorpion protecting him against insect bites. Tattoos might also mark a person as immune from taboos or as having special magical or supernatural powers of his own. In New Guinea tattoos were often dedicated to the spirits of particular parts of the body which were thereby protected and shielded from profane glances. As Frazer has shown, such markings have often been believed to perform a subtle magical function: they put the wearer under the influence and protection of the spirit or totem of the tribe. Though a certain amount of individual freedom was lost thereby, so also was individual responsibility—a not unattractive fate for many people, as Erich Fromm has pointed out. A magical protective mantle was cast over the wearer by the tattoo so that he could forevermore meet with impunity the enemies of war and the evil spirits of the night. Perhaps one of the most remarkable uses of the tattoo, however, was its use as a 'passport' to the next world. Many primitive peoples have believed that 'the ghost fares ill who cannot show his identifying tattoo on his way through the gate to the spirit world.' An equally strange motive, however, was reported by Sumner:

> It was once the great ambition of young men to make themselves conspicuous in war by tattooing, for even if they were killed by the enemy, whilst the heads of the untattooed were treated with indignity and kicked on one side, those which were conspicuous by their beautiful 'moko' were carefully cut off, stuck on the *turuturu,* a pole with a cross on it, and then preserved, all of which was highly gratifying to the survivors, as well as to the spirits of their late possessors.

Opposite *An unusual European example of facial tattooing. Whereas facial pigmentation by tattooing has occasionally been popular among the aristocracy in an effort to counter the grey pallor of old age, other social groups have more often favoured body designs*

4

Sophisticated elaboration

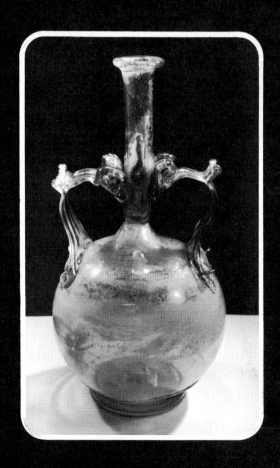

Ovid reassured Roman women in his manual for lovers, the
Ars Amatoria, 'No woman need be ugly, for all the remedies
can be found in pots and potions.' And he gave some useful
recommendations—based mostly on natural substances
such as vetches, beaten barley and egg white—for beautify-
ing the skin. He warned, however, 'Good looks come only
with care, and die if neglected.' His advice to blonde girls
was to 'wear black', 'and if healthy blood cannot colour your
cheeks, rouge will.' Also, if the eyebrows were a little scanty
and time-worn, fresh ones could be glued into position. If
the eyes themselves were not inherently sparkling and
vivacious they might be lined with eye-shadow or saffron.
For Ovid these were serious matters, not to be treated
lightheartedly. He even wrote a poem, the *Medicamina
Faciei,* which contained practical advice on artificial aids to
beauty. It is clear from his writings that a fashionable,
desirable Roman girl at the beginning of the Christian era
would probably have used a good many of these. She would,
according to the current preference, have been tall and
blonde (rather than brunette), worn a plain robe, and had
bright red cheeks and eyes shaded with kohl or painted with
saffron. Her brows would have been pencilled, and she
would have had a patch or two on her cheek or neck, or
perhaps, even more daringly, on her bare shoulder or arm.
Roman men, too, used these cosmetics just like their
womenfolk. Nero, for example, used them liberally; ceruse
and chalk to whiten his face and skin, Egyptian kohl to
blacken his eyes and lashes, and red fucus to brighten his
cheeks and lips. He also used pumice-stone to whiten his
teeth.

In the earliest Roman times there seems to have been
little interest in cosmetics. But increasing concern with the
graces of living followed the Roman migrations to the
south of Italy, a region hitherto occupied by the highly
civilized Greeks. Oils, perfumes and cosmetics soon thereafter became established as important constituents of the
good life, and especially so among the aristocracy. The more
fashionable ladies of the Roman court, using a special soap
imported from Gaul, distinguished themselves by bleaching
their hair to the golden colour so much admired at that time.
In ancient Greece, many coloured substances had been

Opposite *Roman
cosmetic jar*

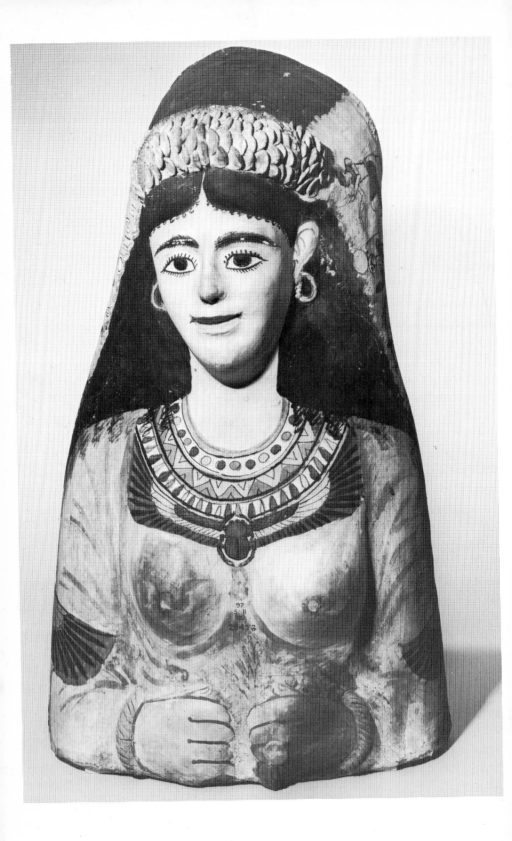

popular for adorning the face—kohl for the eyes, puperissium, a Syrian root, for rouge, and ceruse for whitening.
Since, however, ordinary women were regarded merely as
chattels, the use of such cosmetics was normally reserved
for the men and for courtesans. Their use by courtesans
does not seem to have been specially skilled, since Lucien
recorded, 'If one could see these painted women getting out
of bed one would find them even less attractive than
monkeys.' The Greeks used cosmetics liberally and often
very crudely in their celebrations to the gods and in their
theatrical performances; they used special colours to indicate the identity of different kinds of character. But cosmetics
were used long before the days of Ancient Greece. When
Tutankhamun's tomb was opened in the 1920s, a large
number of cosmetic jars were found—many of them still
retaining, after three thousand years, enough of their sweet
perfume to allow chemical analysis: they contained about
nine parts of animal fat to one of perfumed resin. Many
anthropologists believe that the use of cosmetics derived
originally from the need for protection from sand, insects,
wind and weather. There is evidence that as long as twelve
thousand years ago the Ancient Egyptians were protecting
their bodies and faces with coloured earths and clay and
with grease and oil from the wild castor plant. Soon,
however, they were evidently appreciating and enjoying
the decorative properties of the same substances. Egyptian
records show that some of the first experiments in self-
improvement were made on the eyes: malachite green eye-
paste, for example, originally used to protect the eyes
against light, soon became much prized for its purely
decorative powers. Other coloured substances for the eyes
gradually became popular for use at different times of the
year and in varying light conditions. Cleopatra painted her
upper eyelids blue and her lower eyelids bright green. She
used black kohl to draw in the shape of her eyelids and to
accentuate her eyebrows, and white ceruse for her face,
neck and breasts. She employed yellow ochre to colour her
cheeks, and carmine dyes for her lips. The impulse to
decorate was evidently so strong that when the summer
weather became too hot for impressive displays of rich
clothing the Egyptian courtiers bared their chests, painted

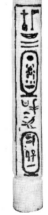

Above *When
Tutankhamun's tomb
was opened in the 1920s
a large number of
cosmetic tubes were
found—including this
tube for kohl eye-
shadow*

Opposite *A canvas
and stucco cover for the
head and chest of a
Roman-Egyptian
Mummy, 1st Century*
AD

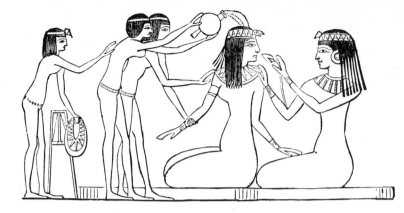

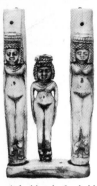

A double tube for kohl decorated with carved relief figures of goddesses and lions. Similar figures appear on the kohl stick-holder in the centre

Top right *An Egyptian lady at her toilet, attended by servants*

Bottom right *Egyptian jars for creams and eye-paints* c. *2000–1500* BC

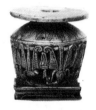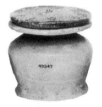

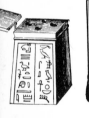

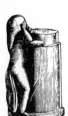

Boxes used by the Ancient Egyptians for eye-paint

their nipples gold and outlined their breast veins in blue.

It was soon realised that much more than physical protection and decoration could be gained by using these coloured substances: they had magical powers too. The spirits of the gods could be invoked by making appropriate markings on the face and body. Much importance was attached to the precise shape, position and colour of these markings, and to the circumstances under which they were applied. If properly made and acquired under the right conditions of ritual and ceremony they could very well protect the wearer against all manner of evils. Originally the priests had developed their pastes, perfumes and chemicals simply for mummification of the dead; they had undertaken a good deal of diligent experimentation and had discovered many genuinely useful chemicals, ointments and creams. They took good care, however, always to encourage and maintain belief in their magical powers by employing them regularly in impressive religious rituals, and by so doing very soon established for themselves a lucrative monopoly industry. This curious belief in the magical powers of cosmetics, and indeed of other forms of facial elaboration, seems to have

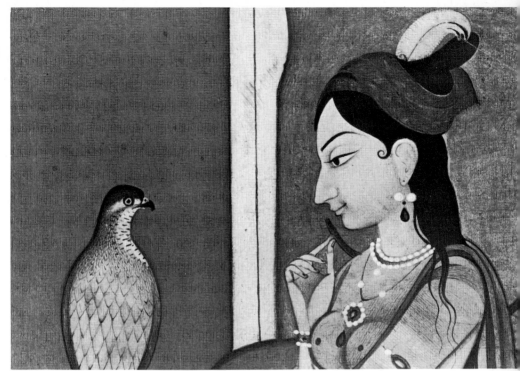

been characteristic of all ages and races; it is widespread even today and skilfully exploited in modern cosmetic advertising.

About a hundred years before Ovid started writing his poems and books of practical advice for Roman lovers, yet another treatise on the arts of love was being compiled by Vatsyayana in a quite different part of the civilised world. This was the *Kama Sutra,* which required that every woman should devote her time entirely to her master and use cosmetics skilfully as one of her 'extra arts' in seduction. Indeed, the perfect Indian woman should be skilled in no less than sixty-four of these 'extra arts'. One of them was 'number 9: colouring the teeth, hair, garments, nails and bodies'. Another was 'number 6: tattooing.'

In the Dark Ages in England, women were mere chattels and beasts of burden. But by the twelfth century their place in society and their share of life's pleasures had improved immeasurably. The Crusaders had returned with various strange Eastern substances—perfumed oils, *eau de Chypre,* dyes for lips and eyes, and strange pastes to whiten the face—all of which were soon to become highly prized.

Above *In India cosmetics have long been used. The* Kama Sutra *required every woman to become skilled in their use as one of her 'extra arts' in seduction. Pahari painting from the Punjab Hills* c. *1750*

Below *Mediaeval elaboration: the Willcotes Effigies in Northleigh Church*

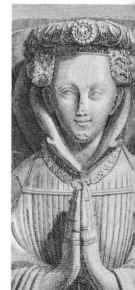

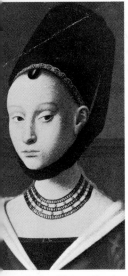

Both in Mediaeval and Elizabethan times the shaved forehead was considered an enhancement to the dignity and the charm of the female face

Left *A young Burgundian lady of 1460. Portrait by Petrus Cristus*

Centre *Mediaeval hairline and ornamentation*

Right *A Florentine lady, 1440*

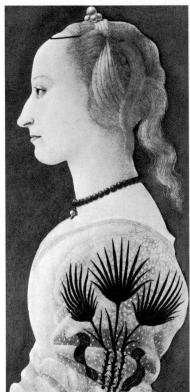

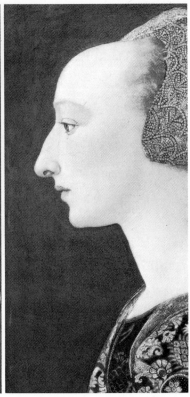

Right *Glenda Jackson's authentic make-up for her BBC portrayal of the ageing Elizabeth I shows the effect of shaved forehead and heavy layers of lead ceruse, popular in the 16th century*

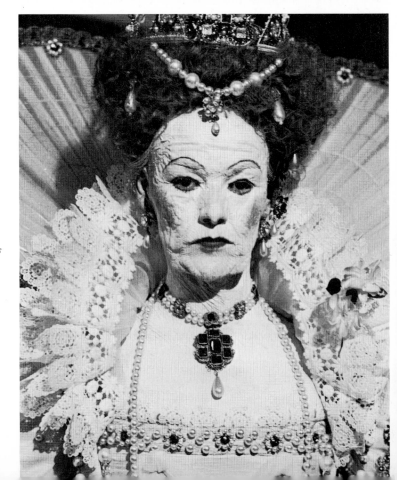

The mediaeval court in England grew suddenly more colourful. At first only the harlots used cosmetics, but soon the ladies too began to wear these paints and pastes in public. At the same time they acquired brighter and more complicated styles of dress. There was altogether much greater concern for personal appearance—encouraged, no doubt, by the metal looking-glasses which had just become available, and perhaps, too, by the beginnings of popular interest in portraiture. By the middle of the twelfth century, many of the fashionable young ladies of England were shaving hair from the front of their heads, and from their eyebrows as well, which gave them a very high forehead. This produced a charming appearance in those with beautiful eyes. Unfortunately it gave plainer women a look of empty stupidity. The remaining hair was often dyed bright crocus yellow. Faces were grotesquely plastered with white paste and lips stained deep red. On the Continent at this time the fashion was rather different: girls were rougeing their cheeks rather than whitening them. One account tells of the cosmetic habits of Isabeau of Bavaria, who became Queen of France in the fourteenth century. Like Cleopatra, she enjoyed bathing in asses' milk. She also used a lotion of boars' brains, crocodile glands and wolves' blood, and other magic lotions and potions produced by the alchemists, confidence tricksters and magicians of her time. All of these substances were liberally applied to her skin to the accompaniment of mystical incantations. After the fourteenth century many books of recipes for such strange and magical beauty concoctions began to appear—and continued to be popular for the next four hundred years.

By the time of Elizabeth I, many tempting and attractive substances had become available for whitening the face and neck, darkening the eyes and reddening the cheeks. One of the most popular was white ceruse, the same substance as had been used by Cleopatra. This was a paste of white lead applied to the skin with a damp cloth. Mixed on a palette; with egg-white and sometimes vinegar, it gave to the face an ethereal whiteness. It was sometimes overlaid with a tinted shellac varnish which must have added yet further immobility to the face. Kohl was also widely used for darkening the eyelids, lashes and eyebrows, just as it had been by the

Ancient Egyptians. Coloured eye-shadows were worn, made from pounded green malachite. A strong mercuric dye, red fucus, was used for the lips. Many of these old cosmetics were in fact highly-dangerous poisons. A cosmetic popular for centuries, for example, for removing freckles, was sublimate of mercury. This not only removed the freckles but stripped away the outer layer of skin and corroded the flesh underneath as well. Many victims of these poisonous substances died at a young age. Perhaps the most notable was the famous beauty Maria Gunning, later the Countess of Coventry, whose death at the early age of twenty-seven was hastened by her continued and obstinate use of ceruse. The addiction of the lovely Countess to lead ceruse and mercuric fucus was such that her husband 'used to chase her round the dinner table that he might remove the obnoxious colour with a napkin.' 'From beef without mustard,' he cried, 'from a servant who over-values himself, and from a woman who painteth herself, Good Lord, deliver us!'

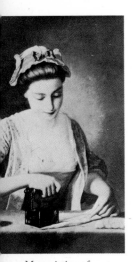

Many victims of cosmetic poisoning died at an early age: Maria Gunning, Countess of Coventry, whose obstinate use of toxic lead-based ceruse hastened her early death at 27. Print, Ironing by H. Morland

Ceruse, popular from Egyptian times until the nineteenth century, was actually composed of lead oxide, hydroxide and carbonate: all deadly cumulative poisons progressively absorbed and stored in the body. Fucus, the popular red lip salve, was made from mercuric sulphide, another deadly poison, which killed many unfortunate women. Other women were made bald in their frantic search for beauty by fearsome applications to their scalp of such noxious substances as sulphuric acid, turmeric and alum water. Kohl, the eye-shadow largely composed of lead and antimony sulphides, was yet another poison.

Abrasives were vigorously applied to the teeth—pumice powder mixed with pounded brick was a particular favourite—and these rapidly removed the enamel along with the stains. It is not surprising that women were reduced to unwholesome wrecks by the time they were thirty. Even children were not immune from these assaults in the name of beauty; their foreheads were covered with walnut oil to decrease the growth of their hair, and their eyebrows were shaved. Painful plasters and quicklime were also used to remove facial hair. How fortunate were the poorer girls who had to be content with cheap cornflour or borax for whitening their faces, and cochineal or berries from the hedgerows for reddening their cheeks and lips.

Face-painting continued to flourish throughout the seventeenth century—so much so that public complaints began to be voiced. The *Spectator* in 1711 protested about the ladies who were known as the 'Painted Picts':

> The muscles of a real face work with soft passions, sudden surprises, and are flushed with agreeable confusions, according as the object before them, or the ideas presented to them, affect their imaginations. But the Picts behold all things with the same air, whether they are joyful or sad, the same fixed insensibility appears on all occasions. A Pict, though she takes all these pains to invite the approach of lovers, is obliged to keep them at a certain distance: a sigh in the languishing lover, if fetched too near, would dissolve a feature; and a kiss snatched by a forward one, might transform the complexion of the mistress to the face of the admirer.

By 1770 Parliament had evidently become so concerned about the enormous variety of cosmetics and artificial aids used by women 'to entrap men into marriage' that an Act was passed imposing the same penalties as were then in force for witchcraft:

> . . . whatever age, rank, profession or degree, whether virgins, maids or widows that shall impose upon, seduce and betray into matrimony any of His Majesty's subjects by the scents, paints, cosmetic washes, artificial teeth, false hair, Spanish wool, iron stays, hoops, high-heeled shoes, bolstered hips, upon conviction the marriage shall be null and void.

This law was, of course, quite unenforceable, and quickly fell into disuse and disrepute. There was nonetheless a decline in the use of cosmetics. By 1784 the *Ladies' Magazine* was reporting that 'white paint is disappearing though a little rouge is very pardonable. White paint is now looked on as disgraceful and dangerous.'

There were no such inhibitions on the Continent, however. Neither the French nor their portrait painters saw any objection to such use of cosmetics, which were soon to reach a high peak of artificiality, in the days of Pompadour, Du Barry and Marie Antoinette. The French felt themselves altogether more advanced and frankly honest about this and

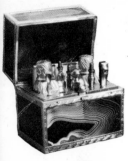

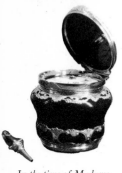

similar matters: prints and paintings of the period show French women in postures which would have been quite unacceptable in polite English portraits—in bed, for example, or at their dressing table, or even at the bidet.

And then, for half a century, between 1790 and 1840, it was the men rather than the women who dominated the cosmetic scene. This was a time of unprecedented effeminacy in men's dress. Beau Brummel was setting new English standards by cleaning his teeth, scrubbing his skin, shaving, and even tweezing out single hairs from his face. He was setting new standards of personal hygiene as stringent as those of the early days of the Roman Empire. After two centuries of such hectic cosmetic dyings and brewings and paintings, the ladies needed a rest.

Regency women, content with fewer and fewer cosmetic aids, were beginning to attract attention to other parts of their bodies by wearing dresses ever more daringly flimsy and revealing. A fashionable dress of the time 'had to be capable of being passed through a wedding ring.' One observer noted 'an alarming increase in pneumonia and bronchitis.' Matters were made worse by the popular habit of wetting the dress so that it might cling more revealingly to the body. During the early part of the nineteenth century, therefore, attention seems to have shifted gradually away from the female face. Ladies relied more and more on clothing and natural aids, such as flowers, to beautify themselves; they used cosmetics only sparingly. A strange and interesting new material known as 'sympathetic blush' or 'Schnouda' made a brief appearance, however. This remarkable substance contained alloxan, a chemical which has the curious property of turning steadily pinker on exposure to air. Skill was needed in its application, since it was difficult to anticipate the final degree of redness which would follow—and many an impulsive user provoked much amusement and scorn as the evening progressed and her face glowed increasingly bright with blotches of ever-deepening red.

By the time Victoria was on the throne, the use of cosmetics had virtually disappeared—the only beauty aid allowed in polite Victorian society being a discreet dash of eau de Cologne. Rouge and face paints were judged quite improper. The Victorian lady of fashion retreated from the

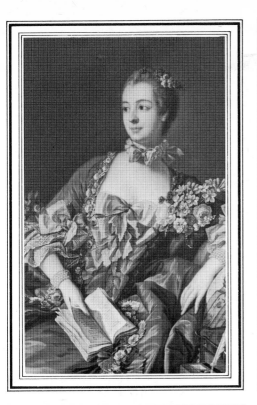

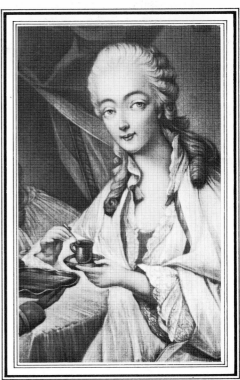

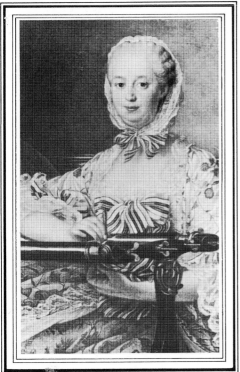

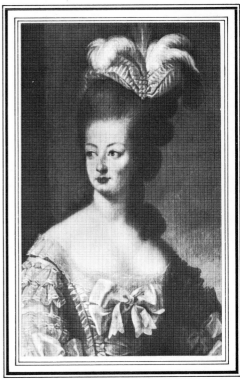

The Victorian *attitude: cleanliness, the only way to beauty. Advertisement,* The Graphic *Jan. 19, 1889*

Right & below: In the late 19th century cosmetics had fallen out of favour: artificial aids to beauty were considered 'immoral' and could only be advertised by masquerading as healers

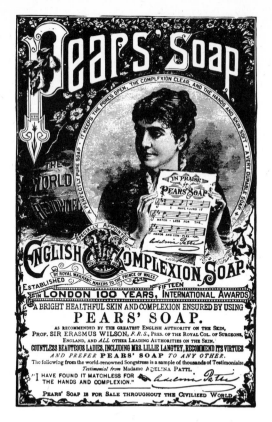

Oyez! Oyez! Oyez!

yͤ Earlie Englyſhe Soape,

ESTABLYSHED 100 YEARS,

Pears' Soap,

A Special Preparation for yͤ Complexion:

s uſed and recommended bye *Miſtreſs Adelina Patti, Miſtreſs Lillie Langtry,* **and** othere beauteous Ladyes. Yͤ Soape is marvellous for improving yͤ Complexyon, and for keepynge yͤ handes inne nice ordere. Yͤ Proprietors of PEARS' SOAP are yͤ makers bye Royal Warraunt to yͤ 𝔓𝔯𝔦𝔫𝔠𝔢 𝔬𝔣 𝔚𝔞𝔩𝔢𝔰,

All yͤ Dealers sell it.

harsh light of day, relaxed on her couch, and showed herself as little as possible. For shopping she took cover under a bonnet, sometimes even a veil. Her pallor was so acute it was sometimes described as 'the green sickness'. The ideal Victorian beauty, whose virtues were so extolled by novelists and poets, had a small roseate mouth, her eyes were large and deep blue, shining under beautiful arched brows. Her skin however, had to be deathly pale.

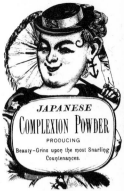

But although the Victorian lady had almost relinquished cosmetic aids by the mid-nineteenth century the English gentleman's toilet armoury was still likely to be considerable. It would include perfumed chalk if he were too florid, or rouge if too pale. Castor oil and beeswax he would have too, for promoting the growth and health of his hair, and tweezers for removing unwanted eyebrows. Even as late as 1877 Lord Malmesbury was skilfully rouged, as Disraeli records:

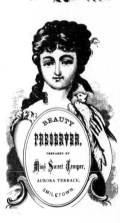

> People say that resource to cosmetics is effeminate but Malmesbury is manly enough, and the two most manly persons I ever knew, Palmerston and Lyndhurst, both rouged. So one must not trust too much to general observation.

It was not until the end of Victoria's reign that female cosmetics were allowed to return, and even then they were obliged to masquerade as healers. In 1886, Harriet Hubbard Ayer offered for sale a cream whose formula was said to have been handed down from Julie Recamier, celebrated for forty years or more as 'the most beautiful woman in France.' But adverse attitudes towards cosmetics were so entrenched that the cream could be offered for sale only as a 'healer for removing spots'. Helena Rubinstein, too, concentrated on the medicated properties of her first 'Valaze' cream, later to be described as 'Skin Cleansing Cream'. Elizabeth Arden laid careful stress in her advertising at that time, on the need for good general health and physical fitness if a beautiful complexion were to be achieved. Her products were offered to do no more than aid and encourage nature. Victorian advertising was extremely cautious: any artificial aid to beauty, even perhaps beauty itself, was still not quite respectable. Cheeseborough Ponds developed the popularity of Ponds Extract Cream by describing it first and foremost

Facial masks in use at a Beauty School in the USA

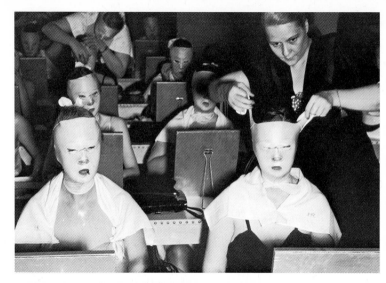

Left *The 20th century attitude: every device of science and medicine must be mobilised in the pursuit of beauty. Equipment for facial massage*

Right *A facial mud-pack at the Austrian Spa of Neydharting where the local mud is reputed to have medicinal qualities*

Right & opposite: *Modern make-up (including 'the costliest perfume in the world')*

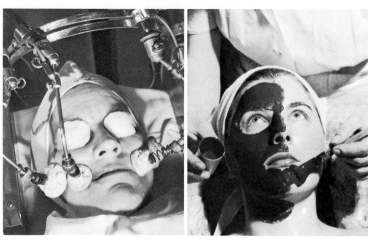

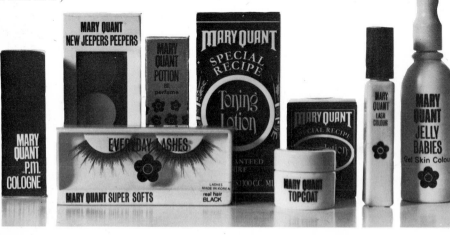

as being good for 'constipation, colds in the head, hay fever, malarial fever, syphilis and typhoid'. It also happened to be good for the face, and Harriet Ayer wrote a little booklet on its healing qualities, giving instructions for a 'cream bath', whose purpose was of course simply to 'cleanse' the skin—certainly not to adorn it.

The history of the advertising of cosmetics is interesting not only because it reflects the attitudes of the time but also because it provides us with valuable indirect evidence about the psychological motivations underlying facial adornment. There seems to be in all peoples, sophisticated as well as primitive, a strong need for mystery, magic and ritual. It is a need which has been well satisfied for thousands of years by the mystical rituals accompanying facial decoration. Even today, advertisers often suggest by their brand names that their products offer not only physical enhancement but magical protection. A careful ritual must be precisely followed in their application. And nowadays additional magic is provided in the form of science and medicine: new technological miracles are available—hypo-allergenic preparations for ultra-sensitive skins, hormones for magical youth, powerful new 'bio-energetic' formulae, and much more besides. Even the potent, fertile mysteries of the queen bee have been mobilised by modern science to add lustre and delight to the skin. Many products also offer, just as the ancient ones did, an opportunity for sacrifice. Many modern 'mud packs' and 'treatments' are not pleasant—though none perhaps is nearly so unpleasant as the crocodile dung used as a 'face-pack' in ancient Rome. These new substances extract yet further sacrifice by their high financial cost. The more expensive the product, the more valuable (and effective) it is thought to be. In the early years of the twentieth century, cosmetics had always been expensive and their use was more or less confined to upper-class women. By the end of the First World War, however, cosmetics became cheaper and a new generation of emancipated girls from the ammunition factories were able to buy them, with the result that their over-use became the sign of the worker rather than the upper-class woman. Richer women continued to use them, but in more restrained ways. Superiority was now achieved by the use of products of refined quality

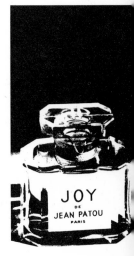

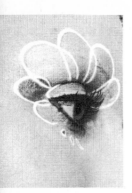

A decorative eye-design by Helena Rubinstein, 1972

and high cost. Even today, many women are prepared to pay £20 for a jar of face-cream; there are also many who find especial delight and satisfaction in 'the most expensive perfume in the world'.

In recent years there has been a much freer and franker recognition in advertising of the sexual role of cosmetics. In the 1930s a picture on the package showing a silhouetted pair of lovers under moonlight and stars was judged a little daring. But nowadays cosmetics are frankly offered as 'man proof' and lipsticks are 'for crushing'. Cosmetics for the face are not enough—'use them on the body—nudity is liberating self-awareness', 'exhibition is fun'. And there is one particular product which 'you can stroke over sensitive areas as often as you like'. 'Scandals', 'Love Affairs' and 'Sins' are fast being overtaken by new freedoms in sexual imagery. But motivational research has at last discovered that the sexual motives are not the strongest spurs to sales. The search for social acceptance and the pursuit of the satisfactions of conformity seem to be much more important motives. Motivational researchers have uncovered, too, an entirely unsuspected inhibition militating against the use of cosmetics: many women, it seems, are more than a little reluctant to think of themselves as the sort of people who are prepared to adopt so much subterfuge and deceit and artificiality. And so advertisers now seek to imply that no real deceit is involved; the purpose of cosmetics is *not* to apply a curtain of pretended beauty but rather to liberate the latent beauty within, by products which 'maximise', 'reveal' and 'make the most of your natural resources'. This is a doubly successful strategy which at once quells the conscience and flatters the user. And today more and more products are sold on their ability to nourish the skin with oils, hormones and even 'moistures' which evidently a parsimonious Nature is not already supplying in sufficient quantity. Nourishing skin foods now go about their work quietly and efficiently in the night; feeding-emulsions coax their way into hungry skin-tissue, complexion milks cleanse, and oils put back muscle-tone into tired flesh—each of them performing a little overnight miracle. The wish to protect and nourish the skin in this way is surely unexceptionable. Surely no guilt can attach to that. And, finally, advertisers

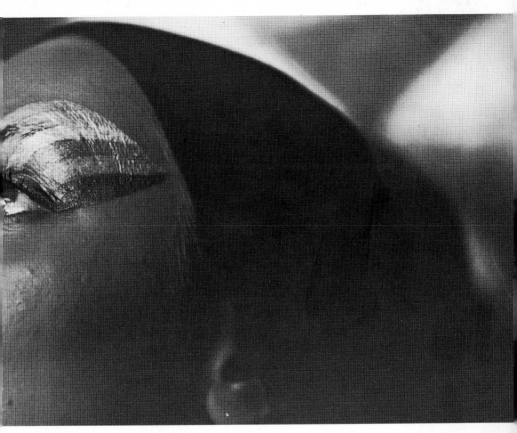

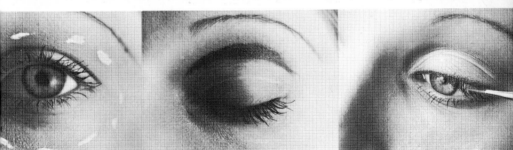

*Modern eye-decoration
by Lancôme*

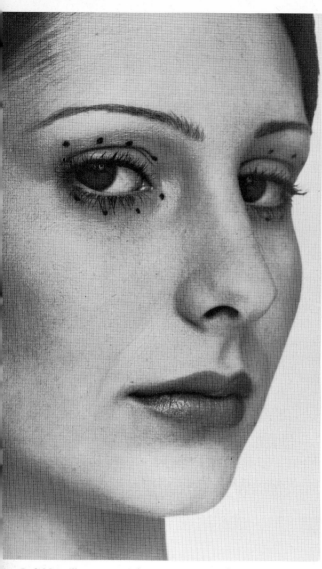 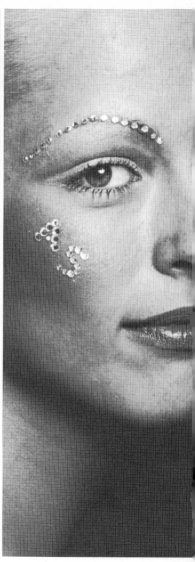

Left Maquillage
Talisman *by Lancôme*

Right *Adele Smith's
party make-up by
Lancôme*

Opposite *Gary Glitter*

have suggested that in any case making-up is just something to be undertaken for fun and harmless pleasure—for the exercise of natural, aesthetic impulses. A disarming streak of humour has also crept into modern advertising, kicking away any last remaining inhibitions. 'Making-up' is now an intelligent, rather sophisticated—perhaps even rather difficult—problem-solving game to be played strictly for our own perfectly proper, narcissistic pleasure and to fit in with the ever-widening range of woman's activities. Cosmetics, after all, are not just for public display. Nowadays, for example, there is even 'Make-up to make love in'.

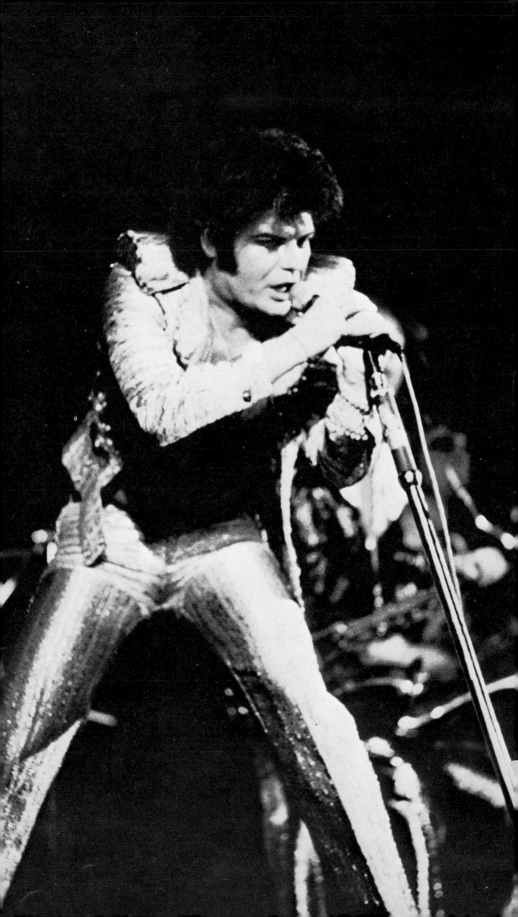

5 Frames for the face

The female face can be adorned in a great variety of ways. Its surface, texture and colour may be improved with creams and powders, its features highlighted by judicious use of specialised cosmetics. Yet there are other, far less obvious, ways of enhancing the total impression. These rely for their effect on the skilful manipulation of the *space around* the face. There are a hundred ways of doing this—by a carefully chosen hairstyle, or wig, or by neck ornaments, or even attractive *décolletage*. Loosely-flowing hair, a gently-moving head-dress, or simply moving ear-pendants may be used to impart a pleasing serenity to the face by the perceptual effect known as 'movement-contrast'. Another contrast effect, that of 'size-contrast', may be used too: a large hat or voluminous *coiffure,* for example, may be used to render the face more petite. It is interesting to discover how, throughout the history of fashion, effects such as these have been intuitively employed in ways which have exaggerated the naturally-occurring differences between female and male. Though there have been many exceptions, female hair and head-dresses have more often been large, and so have even further reduced the apparent size of the female face, already naturally smaller than that of the male. And women have for centuries delighted their admirers with the palest of neckwear and *décolletage*, the effect of which has been to provide the greatest colour contrast imaginable to the dark, hairy jaw and chest of the male. Neck ornamentation, too, with glittering jewellery, has served not only the obvious function of concealing the tired lines and sinewy hollows of the neck but has also provided a bright pale splash of light below the chin, the effect of which is strongly feminine. It is interesting to note, too, that in times when beards were not in fashion and when the male neck was not darkened naturally, men so often chose to clothe their necks and chests in dark and sombre colours.

Perhaps it is the hair, however, which provides the greatest opportunities for providing a flattering frame. Since ancient times, as archaeological remains clearly show, both men and women have lavished much ingenuity and energy on the beautification of their hair. The ancient Egyptians devoted particular attention to their *coiffure;* their hairdressers were highly skilled. Great tiers and tall pyra-

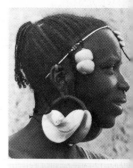
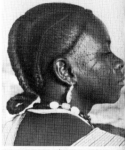
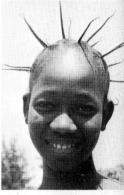

Top *There are few people in the world who can resist the impulse to decorate the space around the face: a Tulah woman from the Upper Niger, 1962*

Middle *The hair provides countless opportunities for decoration: a nomad woman from the Upper Niger, 1962*

Bottom *A student from the Secondary School for Girls in Bamako, Mali, 1964*

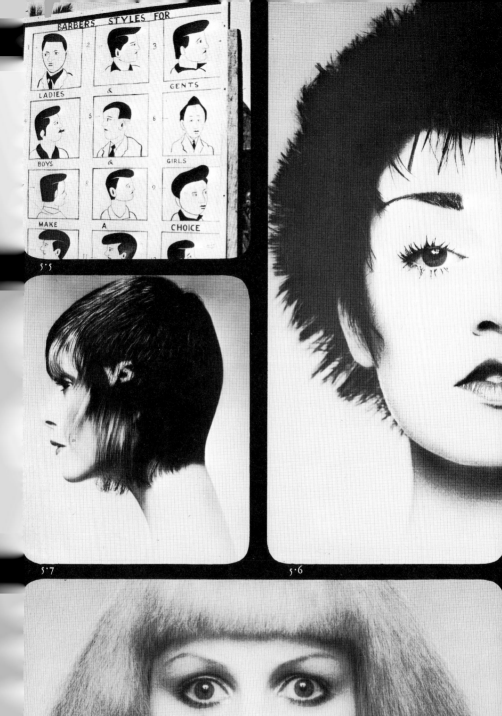

BARBERS STYLES FOR

LADIES & GENTS

BOYS & GIRLS

MAKE A CHOICE

VS

5·5

5·7 5·6

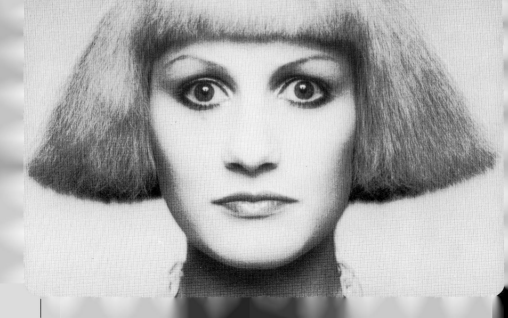

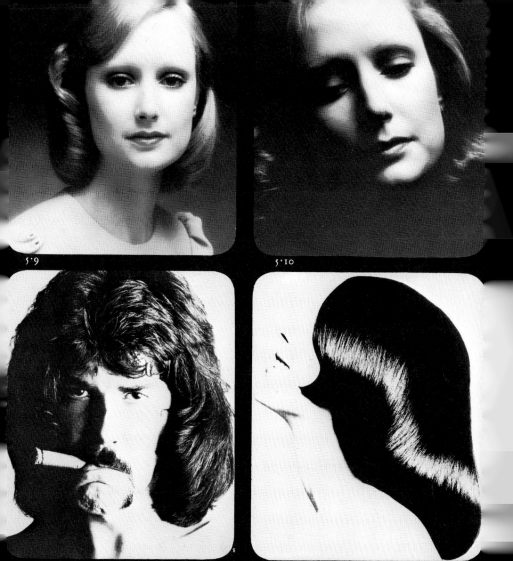

5.9   5.10

5.11   5.12

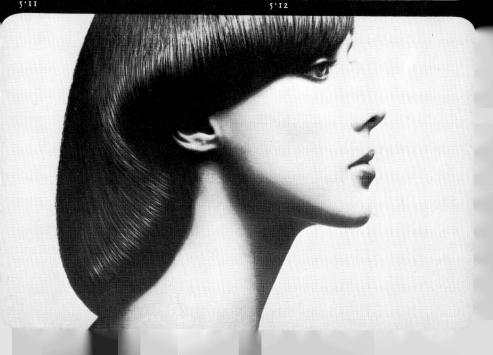

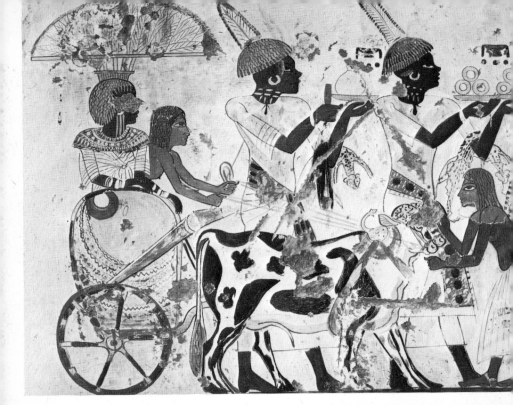

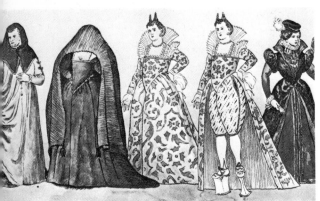

Overleaf:
*Styling is always a
matter of great concern:
a Nigerian barber's
sign, 1962. 5.5
Modern geometric
styles by Vidal Sassoon
'The Brush'. 5.6
'The V.S. Cut'. 5.7
'The Thatch'. 5.8
Hair styling. 5.9/10
Modern hair styling for
males. 5.11
'Isadora'. 5.12
'The Fall'. 5.13*

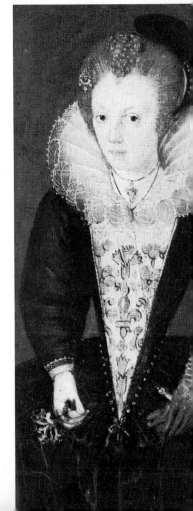

mids of hair were worn by fashionable courtiers, decorated
with all kinds of rich jewellery, and often dyed bright blue,
green or red. The ancient Egyptians were much preoccupied
with the cleanliness of their hair, and frequently used to
insert perfumed balls of wax which slowly melted throughout the day to surround the wearer with a pleasant aroma.
There seems for a time, however, to have been a preference
among the leisured classes for short cropped hair, no doubt
more comfortable in the hot climate. Yet they often chose
to conceal their short hair by wigs of great complexity and
ingenuity. These they used not only in ordinary social
gatherings but in religious ceremonies too, often in special
designs which had particular ritual significance. In Ancient
Greece women wore their hair in long, elaborate styles,
often with many ringlets and rich ornaments of jewels and
gold. Younger men wore their hair short, and often curled,
whereas older Greek men tended to wear their hair long.
There appear to have been many natural blondes in ancient
Greece, who were able, in consequence, to use bright hair
dyes: red and blue and yellow seem to have been especially
popular for festive occasions. Roman women liked to
bleach and dye their hair to bright colours even for everyday wear. It was widely understood that certain dyes, such
as bright yellow, were confined to prostitutes, and consti-
tuted a distinctive mark of their profession.

The ladies of mediaeval times experimented with the
precious hair dyes brought back for the first time from the
Crusades, but they were careful to avoid auburn—the sign
of the witch. During the fourteenth century they developed
a taste for dyed crocus-yellow hair, which continued to be in
fashion until the time of Elizabeth I. During the same century young English women began to pluck and shave the
hair from their hairline, a practice which exaggerated the
height of the forehead and often flattered the features by
reducing their apparent size. Complete plucking of the
brows was also popular and this often produced a striking
effect in a beautiful woman. The raising of the hairline in
this way usually created a youthful, gentle, innocent impression. As Lorenz has recently demonstrated, a large
forehead reminds us of the tenderness of young babies,
whose foreheads are proportionately very large. In Eliza-

Frames for the face

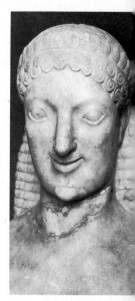

Above *In Greek and
Roman times highly-
formalised hair designs
were much admired.
L'Apollo Milani
(Greek, 525 BC)*

Opposite:
Top *Geometrical hair-
styling 3,000 years ago:
wall painting of the
tomb of Huy, a
contemporary of
Tutankhamun*

Left *Venetian fashions
1600: a variety of
frames for the face*

Right *Ruffs and hair
ornamentation: in
Elizabethan times the
alteration of facial
proportions by shaving
the forehead led people
to search for new ways
of framing the face*

Right
This Baroque portrait bust of Charles II by Honoré Pelle shows the magnificence achieved by the wig even before its heyday in the 18th century

Below
By the end of the 17th century highly decorated hairstyles of great magnificence and complexity had become popular. This wax-effigy in Westminster Abbey shows the elaborately-ribboned hair of the Duchess of Richmond (d. 1702)

Middle
Throughout the 18th century hairstyles and millinery were of great complexity.
Bottom *Bonnet au Pouf*
Top *Bonnet à la paysanne*

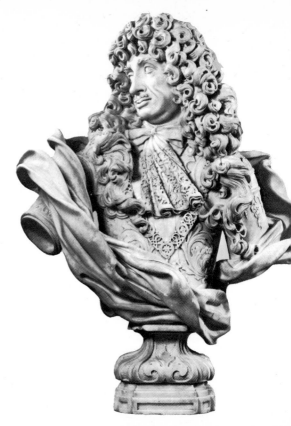

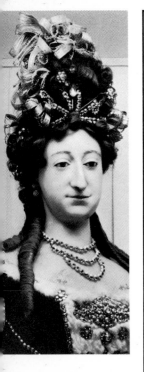

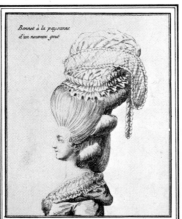

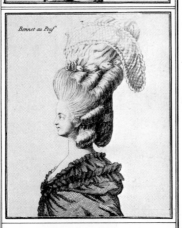

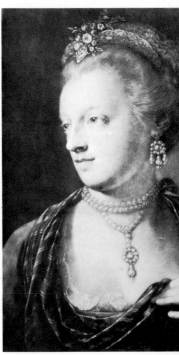

beth's time, the *royal* auburn became fashionable, and crocus-yellow declined in popularity. Even the menfolk began to dye their beards orange. There was also a masculine fashion, in Elizabeth's time, for the lovelock, a curl of hair over the forehead adjusted periodically, with great care, with the aid of a small mirror carried in the hat especially for the purpose. But soon after Elizabeth's death, golden hair again came into favour, and there followed a period of strange and wild excesses: the hair was even gilded and fixed into elaborate designs with gum and honey. The most popular cosmetic was ceruse which not only irritated the skin but also corroded the hair at the hair-line. Once again it became necessary, as well as fashionable, to shave the front hair, as in mediaeval times.

Cromwellian austerity discouraged all forms of ostentation, and long hair for men became unfashionable. Following the Restoration, however, there was a rapid return to the longer 'more decadent' styles worn by the Cavaliers. And thereafter hair styles became more and more elaborate. In 1680, there arose a fashion for the Hurluberlu—an attractive mass of curls worn close to the head. And just before the end of the seventeenth century there was a great upsurge of interest in *coiffure,* and elaborate styles were eagerly sought. Each pattern of curls acquired its own attractive French title to describe its special character: 'Bergères', for example, or 'Favorites', or 'Confidants', or the popular 'Crève Coeurs'. Even Hogarth, who, above all else, considered simplicity the highest attribute of beauty, gave his blessing to this elaborate dressing of the hair. In his *Treatise on Beauty* he declared, 'There is no part of the dress which ought to be so much regarded as that of adjusting the hair.' He was careful to give Sarah Malcolm, the condemned Scottish murderess, time to arrange her hair carefully and to rouge her cheeks before he painted her portrait.

The power of the hair to seduce and corrupt men's minds has long been recognised by the Church, which has often required women to conceal its disturbing display. Its total removal in both men and women has often carried religious significance; voluntary removal has often been taken to signify self-sacrifice and devotion. Many writers have gone so far as to suggest that there is a powerful unconscious

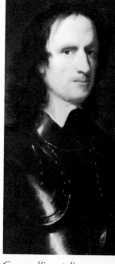

Cromwellian styling

Opposite right
A frame for the face, carefully contrived.
Portrait of a Lady
1761, by T. Frye

association between the hair and sexual activity. Perhaps this explains, in part at least, why preoccupation with the hair is so common. Its length, for example, has always been a source of unending interest and discussion, and has had a number of changing meanings; in some centuries, long hair was the sign of the aristocrat, in others the mark of the peasant or the knave.

As we have seen, women have often been utterly foolhardy in their use of toxic chemicals as facial cosmetics. But they have been even more abandoned in the chemical assaults they have permitted on their hair. The ladies of Venice, according to a writer in 1830, 'used to steep their tresses in caustic solution and sit on their balconies in the sun all day, bleaching it, that the sun might turn it yellow.' In more recent years, harsh chlorine compounds have often been used for bleaching, frequently followed by acidic solutions of cadmium, arsenic or gold in order to impart colour. Arsenic has been used widely for golden hair dyes, usually in the form of orpiment or realgar. Not surprisingly, many deaths have resulted from its use. This passion for poisonous heavy metals has extended even to the choice of accessories: lead combs, for example, enjoyed much popularity because of their capacity, over an extended period of use, to darken the hair. The lead of the combs, when combined with the sulphur in the hair—as well as with traces of sulphur in the atmosphere—produced black lead sulphide, which was gradually deposited in the hair. Another commonly-used poison was oxalic acid:

> Upon one ounce of pure strong oxalic acid, pour a pint of boiling water—and as soon as the hands can bear it, moisten the head thoroughly. If a decided change do not appear at the end of 10 minutes, wet the hair again with the acid, continuing until it affects the skin when it must be discontinued otherwise the hair will fall out.

The impulse to increase the bulk of female hair has often been strong: during the seventeenth and early eighteenth centuries, for example, hair creations of great size and grandeur were worn by ladies of fashion. According to *Sylvia's Book of the Toilet* much discomfort and inconvenience was suffered in consequence:

> Ladies slept in chairs so as not to disarrange their coiffures,

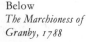

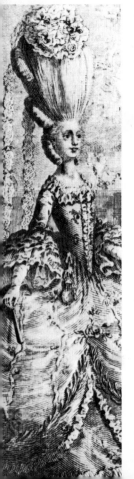

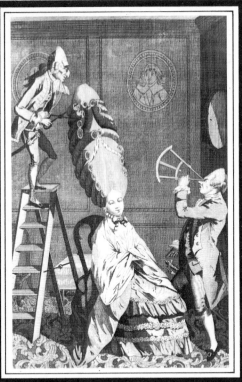

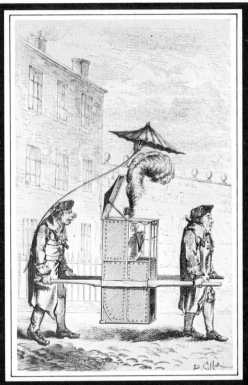

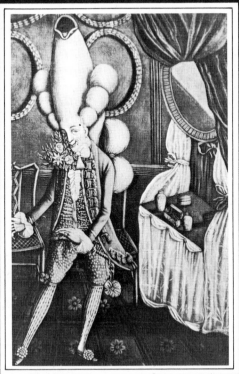

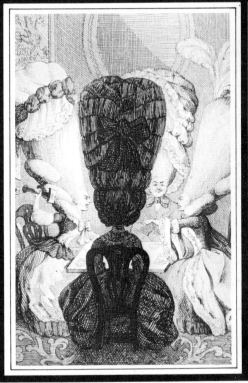

and as 'le galant édifice des cheveux' was so tall as to prevent them from sitting upright in their carriage, they were obliged to kneel during their transit from one house to another.

During the eighteenth century, ladies of fashion often grew their hair long and supported it in grotesque frames reaching three or four feet above their head. Lady Montagu wrote about the ladies of the court of Vienna:

> They build certain fabrics of gauze on their heads, about a yard high, consisting of 3 or 4 storeys, fortified by numberless yards of heavy ribbon. It is considered a particular beauty to have their heads too large to go into a moderate tub. Their hair is prodigiously powdered to conceal the mixture, and set with three or four rows of bodkins, made of diamonds, pearls and red, green and yellow stones.

Often, these monstrous towers of hair were decorated with models of beasts and chariots, or ships in full sail, or perhaps small water bottles like the *boutonnières* used for keeping flowers fresh, or even windmills. Since it was quite impossible to wash these prodigious towers, they very soon became verminous and were made even more offensive, unpleasant and stinking by the decomposition of the flour used for daily dusting in the powder-room.

But there are limits to the development of the bulk in natural hair, and the practical as well as sanitary advantages of an artificial head of hair were becoming increasingly persuasive. Fashion was, by this time, requiring hair in such quantity and complexity of style that it could not be kept clean. Nor was there any great desire to alter a pleasing arrangement once it had been achieved. In consequence the periwig came into favour. Large 'full-bottomed' wigs became popular for men, and somewhat smaller wigs for women. The idea of wigs was not new: they had been used in ancient times by the Medes and the Persians, and by the ancient people of Crete. Xenophon told how the ancient Egyptians wore particularly splendid and ingenious wigs, especially for ceremonial occasions. According to Aristotle, wigs were imported into ancient Greece from Persia, and widely worn by both sexes. They were much used, too, in the Greek theatre. Julius Caesar wore a wig, and the fashionable ladies of the Roman Empire wore bright wigs of many different colours, blonde shades being particular favourites; The wife of Marcus Aurelius was said to have possessed several hundred. Juvenal tells how Messalina, the lascivious wife of Claudius, used wigs as a disguise during her underworld escapades in search of men. The Emperor Caligula similarly found the wig useful as a disguise during his lustings in the town. These Roman wigs were often made from pale hair imported from Germany or shorn from the blonde heads of captured slaves. Some crudely-made 'hair heads' were used in Europe in King Stephen's time, but the wig first came into popular favour in Western Europe after 1624, when the unfortunate young Louis XIII of France suddenly lost both his hair and his beard through illness. Such is the power of Kings that beards promptly ceased to be worn at Court; furthermore, the peruke was immediately adopted by the whole of fashionable society. Soon there were no less than 850 wig-makers in Paris alone —enough to found a Guild of their own. Louis XIV affected a great leonine wig which added inches to his height. It is said that he allowed no man, not even his valet, to see him without it. The fashion spread to England in the time of Charles II though it was denounced as 'devilish' by the Church. Pepys soon found himself experimenting with the new fashion:

> . . . paying £3 for a periwig, tried it out for Church and found it not so strange as I had thought.

Mrs. Pepys, too, found her wig 'pleasant to wear'.

It was in the eighteenth century, however, that wigs achieved their greatest glory. By the time of Queen Anne, they had reached an enormous size, spreading over the chest and covering the back of the shoulders. Walpole described some of the practical difficulties they caused, writing of an interview with Lord Sandwich at the Admiralty:

> I could have no hope of getting at his ear, for he had put on such a first-rate tye-wig that nothing without the lungs of a boatswain can even think to penetrate the curls.

Wigs such as these were built in many different styles and shapes and could cost as much as thirty or forty guineas. They became, in consequence, regular targets for burglars and snatch-thieves. There were many interesting varieties;

copper and iron wire were used to produce 'watch spring' curls in one popular version known as the 'Iron' or 'Wire' wig. All kinds of other substances were used—thread, silk, worsted, mohair, goat's hair and feathers often cunningly combined—and, according to Walpole, 'You wouldn't know it from real hair.' Human hair was used, but it was expensive and might cost as much as £7 for enough for a tied-wig. It was much in demand, however, and poorer women regularly sold their hair for ready cash. Even the peasantry wore short utility wigs, known as 'cut wigs', which were small and neither curled nor powdered. There was a brief revolt against artificial hair in 1765, when many young men suddenly discarded their wigs to the consternation and alarm of the peruke-makers. But this proved only a brief interlude, and wigs soon returned in all their former glory. There were, nevertheless, a number of determined attempts to reduce their cost: the 'Scratch Bob', for example, combined false and natural hair, and covered only the back of the head, the wearer's hair being brought up and brushed over the wig to which it was attached by pomatum. It was a great favourite of horsemen and parsons. And, just as had happened with beards in the sixteenth century, particular styles and shapes came to be associated with each profession: doctors, barristers, parsons and soldiers became easily recognisable from the cut of their wig. Fielding, in one of

An assortment of wig designs. Engraving by Hogarth

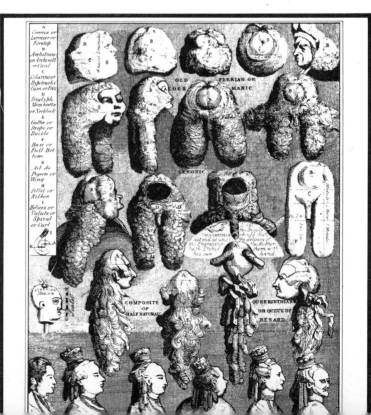

his farces, makes his 'mock doctor' say, 'I must have a physician's habit, for a physician can no more prescribe without a full wig than without a fee.' Even different regiments adopted different styles and colours for powdering their wigs—the 'Buffs' and the 'Blues', for example, each using their own distinctive powders. 'Powder Blue' has persisted to the present day as a colour designation. Pitt is often said to have killed the wig when he introduced a tax of a guinea a year on the use of hair powder in 1795. A few professional groups such as lawyers were exempted, but the remainder, who had to pay, were mockingly described as the 'guinea pigs'. Unlike some other laws of the period, this particular rule was rigidly enforced, and there are many records of the fining of offenders. Thereafter the decline was swift: by the end of George III's reign, few wigs were being worn in England. In France the end was even more abrupt, for after 1789 the wig had become the hated symbol of the aristocracy.

For a while, the wig became simply the distinguishing mark of the doctor, the lawyer and the cleric. However, by Queen Victoria's Coronation the only cleric who wore a wig was the Archbishop of Canterbury, and to this day the ceremonial wig has become limited in Britain to barristers, judges and speakers of the House of Commons.

Wigs of many kinds have become very popular again in

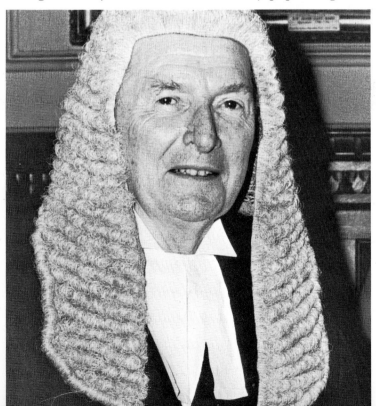

Mr. Speaker: The Rt. Hon. Selwyn Lloyd, MP

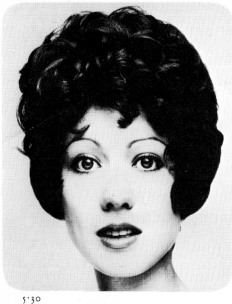

5·30

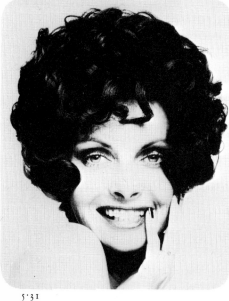

5·31

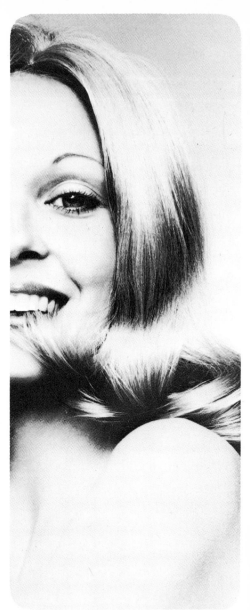

5·32

The effect of wigs: two different wigs are here worn by one model and three by another

recent years, and have gained wide acceptance as purely ornamental devices. They make no pretence to naturalness. Some of them, the more expensive, are made of real hair, whereas others are made from nylon or other artificial fibres. They have many advantages over the wigs of former times: they can be shampooed and set and even permanently waved, and, like cosmetics, can be chosen to suit the occasion. Their colours are unlimited; they may be blonde,

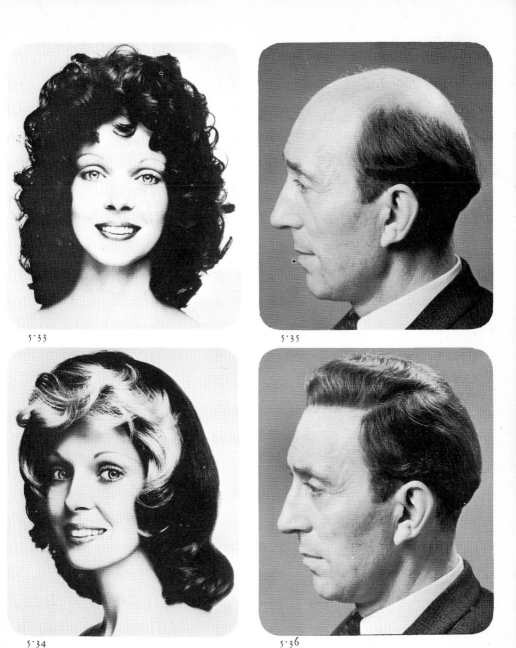

5·33

5·35

5·34

5·36

auburn or gold, but they might equally well be blue. Toupées for men have also become increasingly popular since
the beginning of this century. The male wig industry has
grown very rapidly in recent years. One authority has
estimated that more than a million American men are today
wearing a hairpiece—which is witness enough to the deep
emotional significance of the hair.

It is indeed curious why men themselves should attach

*Modern, well-made
wigs are undetectable*

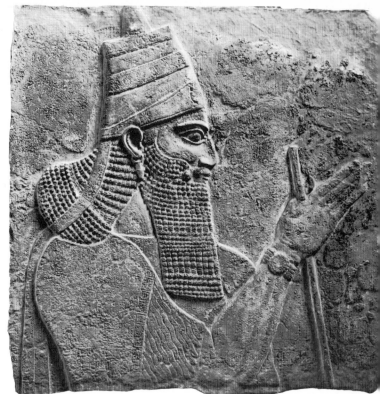

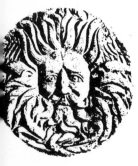

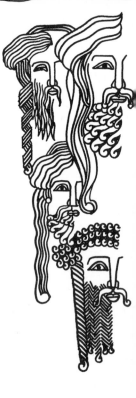

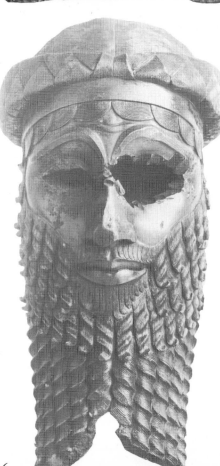

Top *In ancient Assyria
beards were made firm
and stiff by perfumed
gum and resin: a relief
of King Tiglath (1745–
1727 BC) from
Nimrud*

Left *Medusa Mask*

Middle *Sargon, an
ancient Akkadian ruler
of Mesopotamia*

Right *Indian bearded
Bacchus after Thomas
Hope* Costume of the
Ancients

such importance to their receding hair-line when they have at their disposal for display that profoundly male appendage, the beard. An old Maori proverb declares 'There's no woman for a hairy man.' But the history of the beard hardly bears this out. There is, in fact, convincing evidence that the beard has been widely regarded since antiquity as a badge of virility and strength. It was much cherished, for example, by the ancient Babylonians, as a sign of manhood. They lavished great care on their beards, decorating them with rows of elegant curls and making them stiff with perfumed gum. In ancient Greece there was evidently a similar senti-ment: Diogenes is said to have enjoyed taunting his clean-shaven breathren with the cry, 'What sex are you?' Among the ancient Hebrews the beard was valued both as a sign of strength and as a mark of wisdom and enlightenment. Jehovah and his prophets, and Noah too, were invariably described and represented as bearded, and Adam was always depicted in early paintings complete with beard. The Old Testament counselled all good men:

Ye shall not round the corners of your heads, neither shalt thou mar the corners of thy beard. (*Leviticus* 19:27). To the Assyrians and the Ancient Egyptians, the beard was the sign of social rank and sometimes even of divinity. In the temples of the Nile Valley the gods are still to be seen, in sculpture and bas-relief, wearing their special distinguishing mark, the plaited beard. Tutankamun's golden mask had such a beard, since he was considered divine. All but the nobility of ancient Egypt were clean shaven: the beard was the unchallenged prerogative of rulers. The upper classes often chose to wear artificial rather than real beards—in graded sizes to denote social rank. Queen Matshrtpdont wore such a false ceremonial beard, appropriately gilded and jewelled, to mark her authority and majesty. But a curious exception was made to the rule restricting beards to the nobility: commoners in mourning were allowed to grow real beards or, if they wished, to wear false ones.

The early Greeks valued the beard, and particularly the white beard, as a sign of wisdom and authority. Socrates was reverently described by his contemporaries as 'the bearded master'. And there was more than a little preoccu-pation with the beard in Greek mythology: the great Zeus

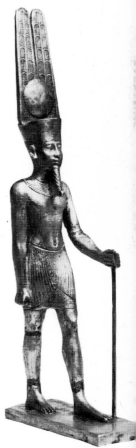

A gold-plated silver figure of Amun-Re (XXII Dynasty). His plaited beard was a sign of his divinity

himself was always portrayed bearded. There was even a legend about Dionysus stealing the gold whiskers of Aesculapius, patron of doctors and barbers, and thereafter fearing to be shaved lest quick vengeance be taken on him. There was also a curious custom in Greece of touching the beard of the man from whom you were seeking a favour. But in other lands, and at other times, the beard has more often been considered sacred, something to be sworn by, like the beard of Mohammed, but never to be touched. Several folk legends tell of babies being put to death for daring to touch their own father's beard. Interference with the beard has often been accounted the ultimate humiliation, and there are many tales of victorious conquerors contemptuously weaving mats from the beards of the vanquished. David went to war to avenge the indignity suffered when his peaceful emissaries had their beards clipped by the Ammonites, who had suspected they were spies. King John inflicted what was considered at the time the highest possible humiliation on the Irish insurrectionists by cutting off their beards; he succeeded only in inflaming their passions irretrievably. And Drake's magnificent exploit at Cadiz could not have been more highly rejoiced in, nor more aptly styled in its day, than as a 'singeing of Philip's beard.' The mediaeval Kings Henry II and Edward III wore long beards, and up to the middle of the fifteenth century most men in Europe were bearded. Then came a beardless interlude; all the English Kings from Henry V to Henry VIII were clean-shaven. Henry VIII required his courtiers to grow short, crisp 'Holbein' beards. But in spite of this royal support the beard encountered a good deal of official opposition. In the last years of the sixteenth century bearded lawyers were charged extra fees to take dinners in their Inns of Court. The young Edward VI even tried to impose a tax on beards, but without success. This was only the first of many such unsuccessful attempts; Elizabeth I tried and also failed. In Russia, Peter the Great tried to tax beards in 1705 and almost provoked a rebellion. In 1722 another attempt was made and the Russian Law was stiffened: if a beard was worn then special clothes also had to be worn and a special tax paid. Catherine I continued and extended this prohibition, but Catherine II gave up the attempt as hopeless and per-

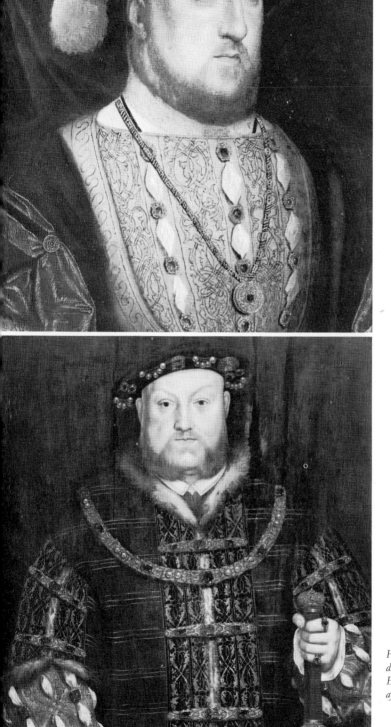

Henry VIII reintroduced the beard into England. Portraits after Holbein

mitted beards to be worn again throughout Russia.

Gentlemen of Elizabeth's time lavished much care on their beards, spreading oils, pomades and perfumes on them, and shaping them in distinctive ways. Shapes became specialised and acquired attractive names such as 'the Dutch', 'the Italian', 'the Court', 'the Country', 'the Old' and 'the New'. A man's profession became instantly recognisable from the cut of his beard—the clergyman from his long 'Cathedral', the soldier from his 'Spade'. The Puritans heartily disapproved, and steadfastly remained clean-shaven. After the Restoration of Charles II, however, the wig began to be increasingly popular. It is curious to discover that at just this time the beard began to decline in favour. There does seem, indeed, to be an antipathy between wigs and beards. It is interesting to find from a careful study of old portraits how the wig and the beard are never to be seen gracing the same face. The beard was destined to remain out of favour for no less than two hundred years: from the middle of the seventeenth century until well into the nineteenth century the majority of men in Europe were clean-shaven.

But in America it was a different story. Leif Ericson, Eric the Red and Columbus were all bearded. So were the Jamestown colonists. In fact the first beardless men in America were the Pilgrim Fathers. Even during the eighteenth century, when shaving had been adopted by the whole of the rest of the civilised world, American men persisted with their beards. Yet by 1830 a strong feeling had somehow arisen against beards. One man at least, John Palmer of Leominster, Massachusetts, determined to please himself, was, in consequence 'Thrown into prison', as his tombstone testifies, 'for wearing a beard.' Many men in the past have fought proudly to retain their beards. A French churchman, Duprat, even resigned his Bishopric rather than give up his beard. Sir Thomas More expressed great concern for his beard at his execution block, brushing it gently aside as he said, '. . . my beard has not been guilty of treason. It were an injustice to punish it.' Later in the nineteenth century, the beard began to return. First of all, sideburns began to appear—named after the American General Burnside. Then came 'muttonchops', 'Picca-

Opposite:
Over the centuries masculinity has been proclaimed by a great variety of beards and moustaches

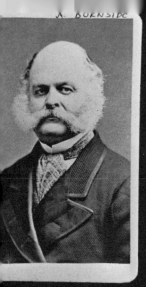

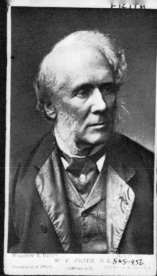

Window & Grove W. P. FRITH, R.A. 845-1956
Permanent Phot. COPYRIGHT.

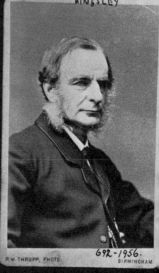

R.W. THRUPP, PHOTO 692-1956. BIRMINGHAM

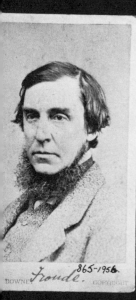

DOWNEY Froude 865-1956 COPYRIGHT

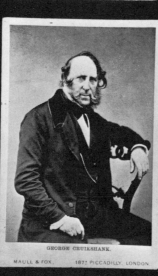

GEORGE CRUIKSHANK.
MAULL & FOX, 187? PICCADILLY, LONDON

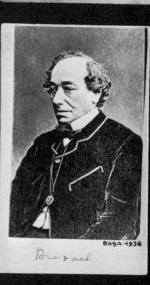

Disraeli 8090-1938

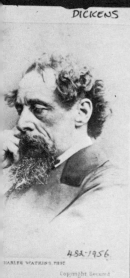

482-1956
CHARLES WATKINS, PHOT
Copyright Secured

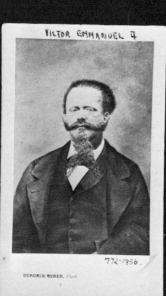

772-1956.
DURONI & MURER, Phot.

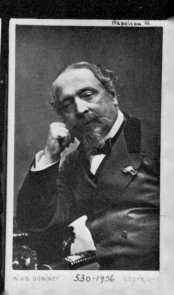

W & D. DOWNEY 530-1956 COPYRIGHT

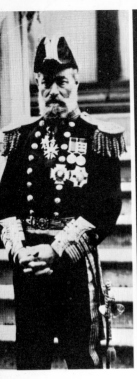

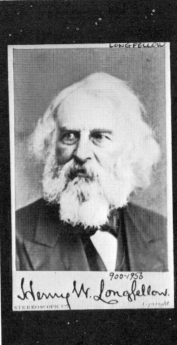

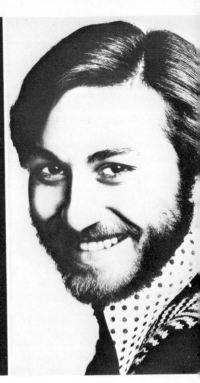

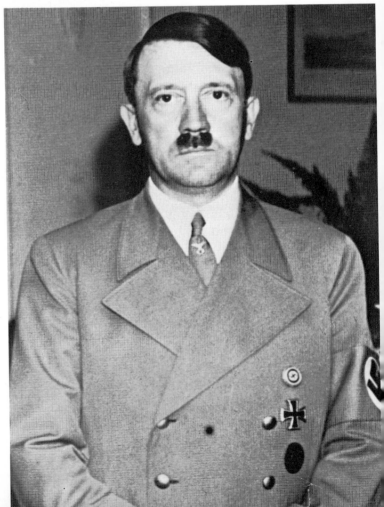

Above:
Left *Traditional naval beard*

Middle *Henry W. Longfellow*

Right *Seventies style*

Right *Adolph Hitler recognised the importance, for a political figure, of simple, easily-remembered, personal marks of distinction. He successfully exploited the infamous trio of moustache, forelock and salute*

dilly weepers', and the 'Dundreary'. Napoleon III's 'Imperial' followed later. During the American Civil War the 'goatee' of the Southern Colonels became popular. Large, luxuriant beards began to be worn by the soldiers—as, for example, by General Grant, the first of a long line of American Presidents to wear a beard. It was McKinley who broke the tradition: since his time all but one of the Presidents of America have been clean-shaven.

In Europe, the crisis of the Crimean War provided the final excuse, if such were needed, for the growth of full beards 'as protection against neuralgia' from the bitter cold of the Crimea. The beard suggested military participation and became fashionably patriotic. It is curious to discover how doctors have often prescribed the wearing of beards as a cure for throat complaints and sometimes, like Adrian James, the sixteenth-century physician, for several other physical ailments besides. As in the present century, however, it was noticeably the poets, artists, and reformers who were the first to reintroduce the beard in the nineteenth century. Beards too were notable among musicians. The pianist Chopin wore a highly eccentric beard—on one side only of his face. 'It does not matter', he said, 'My audience see only my right side.' There were many curious fads, like the sudden craze for bright red beards in 1855—and for the huge walrus moustache some years later. By the nineties, however, the beard seemed to be losing much of its charm; it succumbed easily to the revolt of young intellectuals like Max Beerbohm, Oscar Wilde and Aubrey Beardsley, who appeared in public aggressively clean-shaven. By 1910, all but older men were clean-shaven, although moustaches continued to be worn in the Army and the Royal Air Force and full beards in the Royal Navy.

Below Mark Twain

Bottom right Charlie Chaplin

Bottom left A 19th century advertisement for moustache-setting fluid

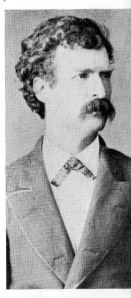

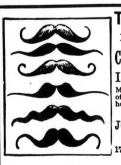
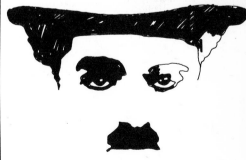

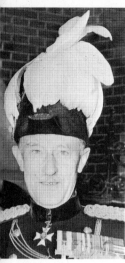

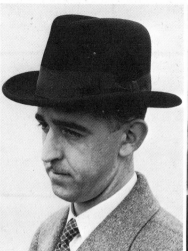

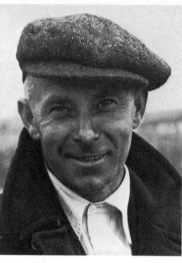

But there is another important opportunity for framing the face not yet considered here: the hat. This can be one of the most powerful elements in the framing of the face. It can flatter, change the mood, even alter the apparent size and proportions of the face as well as providing physical protection. Head-dress has often played an important part in social life and in religious ritual and ceremonial. It serves to indicate to everyone the social structure of a complex, perhaps confusing, human gathering; it marks out the individuals of special rank and status; it defines the *dramatis personae* of today's event. Clear definition of roles is essential to the smooth running of any human or animal community; each member must have a clearly appointed place so that he can be reasonably secure in the knowledge that he will not be challenged or disturbed provided he obeys the rules appropriate to his status. Hats have often done great service as badges of rank and status. The top hat and the cloth cap, for example, each had clear social implications—and there were always strong social pressures against infringements of the rules governing their use. Keir Hardy's appearance in the House of Commons in a cloth cap scandalised his fellow members and, indeed, the country at large. And only when Edward, Prince of Wales, 'sanctioned' the Homburg could it be worn in polite society in place of the hitherto mandatory top hat. The soft felt 'Trilby' similarly had to wait for royal approval before it could be worn generally. Even the colours of hats were subject to similar restriction:

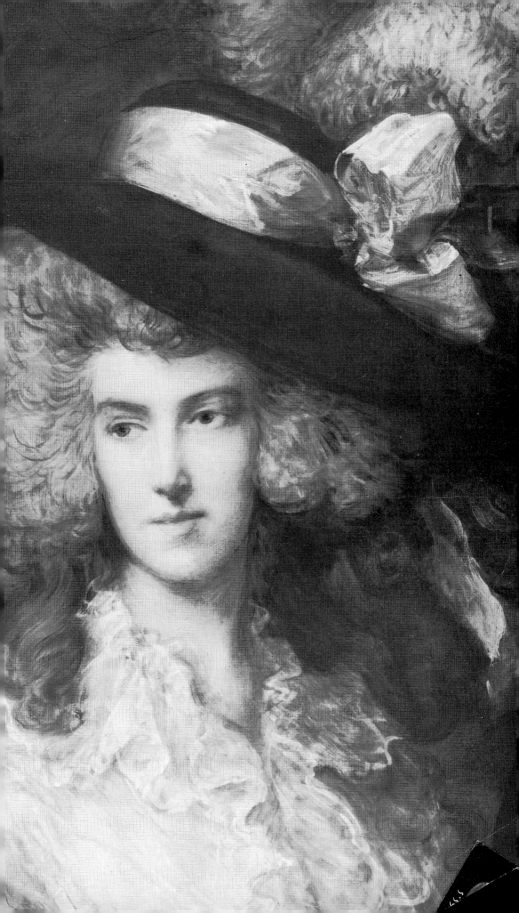

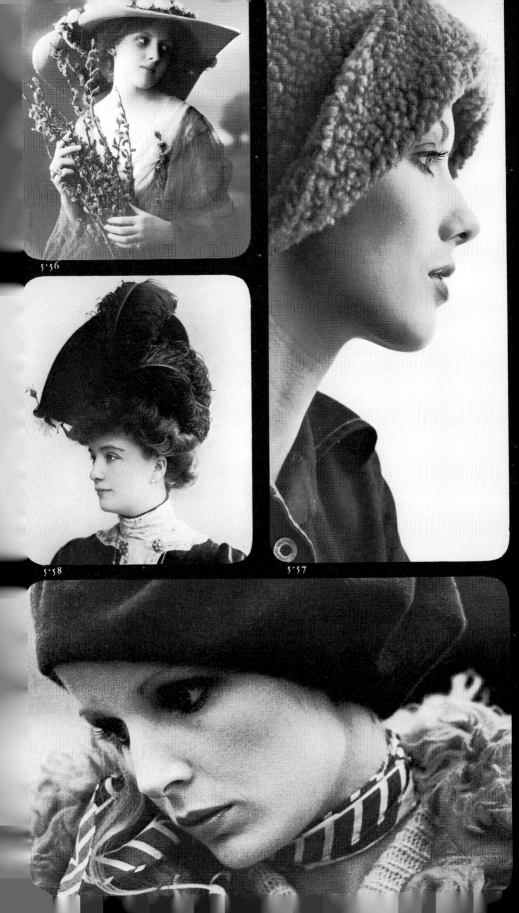

5·56

5·58   5·57

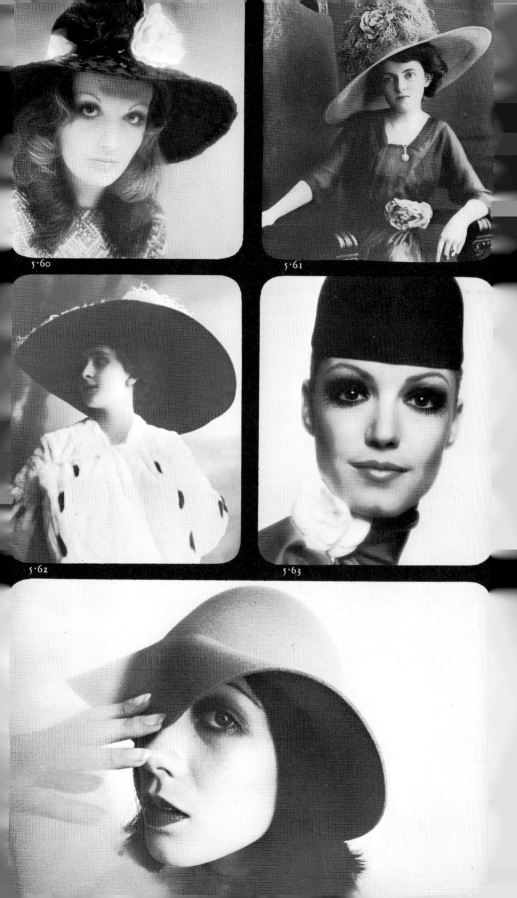

5·60

5·61

5·62

5·63

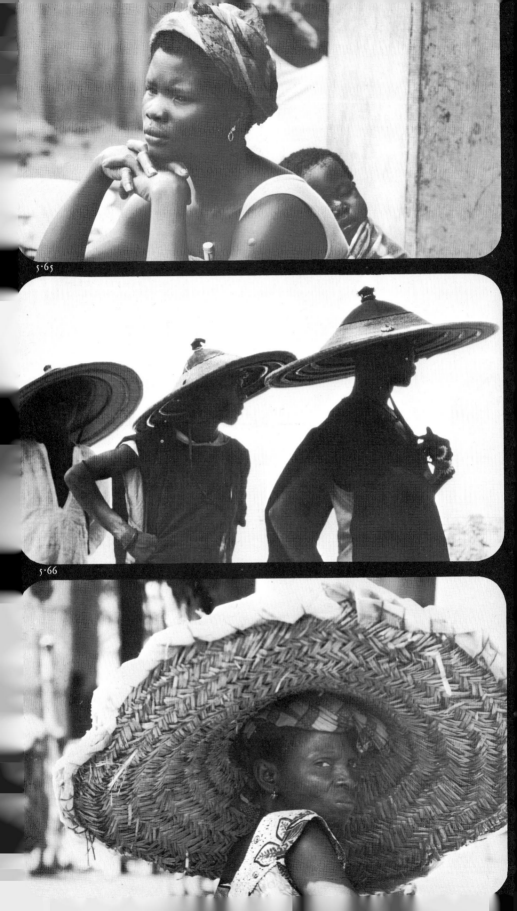

5·65

5·66

Lady Troubridge in her book on etiquette advised that
brown was 'good enough for bookies but not for gentlemen.' It should 'never be worn in London unless you wish
to earn the sneer of the footman.'

As well as adding height and dignity to the wearer, a
large head-dress often reduces the apparent size of a face.
This frequently has a pleasing effect, particularly in a female.
By contrast, a small, close-fitting hat accentuates the size of
the face. Though small hats are often enhancing for men
there are few women fortunate enough to benefit from such
highlighting. The universal flatterer for women, the large
brimmed hat, may enhance attractiveness in another way;
the gentle movements of its brim may impart a feminine
placidity to the face. Again, it may tantalise the admirer by
occasionally concealing parts of the face. Many hoods and
bonnets owe their attractiveness to such occasional concealment. But there are, as we shall see, many other devices
for achieving partial facial concealment. Some of these have
enjoyed considerable popularity and, as our illustration
shows, even *total* facial concealment has sometimes been
fashionable.

Frames for the face

Overleaf left:
Edwardian millinery
5.56/58/61/62
Millinery of the seventies.
5.57/59/60/63/64

Opposite:
Top *Ivory Coast, 1969*

Middle *Boys wearing
straw hats in the San Po
river region of West
Africa, 1962*

Bottom *Abidjan
market*

Below *Total conceal-
ment: a Japanese lady
of quality in Nagasaki.
An engraving from
Ambassades Memor-
ables by Arnoldus
Montanus*

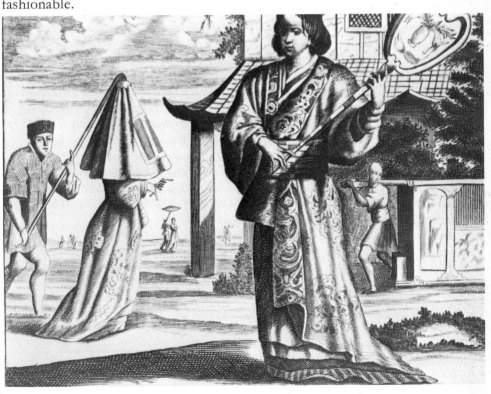

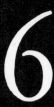

Artful concealment

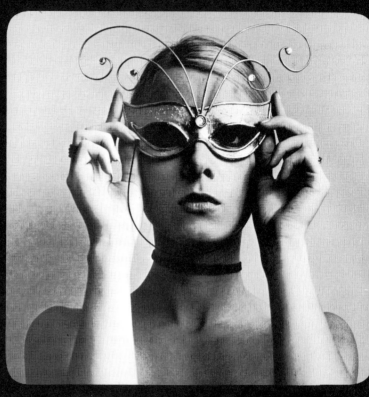

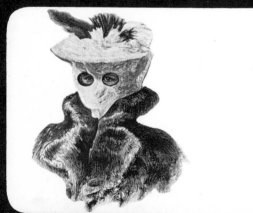

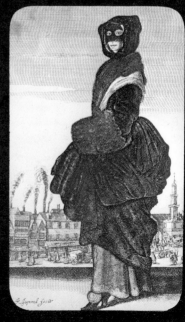

The ladies of the sixteenth and seventeenth century concealed their faces with small masks which had the added advantage of covering up the ravages of disease and caustic cosmetics. They were a great comfort, too, when riding out in cold winter weather. The fact, however, that they were worn in towns much more than in the country suggests that their true function was not so much physical as psychological; they added a pleasing piquancy to social gatherings and became an amusing device of coquetry. And as London's pleasure gardens at Vauxhall became increasingly popular as a place of democratic gathering, the mask acquired something of the character of a uniform for the genteel of both sexes—something which had to be worn to secure anonymity and yet to assert one's social status. The paintings of Guardi show how in Venice also, during the eighteenth century, the mask became part of the uniform of the aristocrat. In America in the eighteenth century, masks were, for a time, required dress for riding. For grown girls and young ladies these riding masks were often made of green silk; younger girls had to be content with white linen. The white linen versions were fastened securely with strings beneath the hood, so that there would be no temptation to employ them in coquettish games. For adults, however, rich, highly-coloured materials were often used to make them: satins, velvets and taffetas, with silk or soft leather for linings. Some were held in place by a silver or bone stud gripped between the teeth. Whatever else this may have achieved it must have given its female wearer a pleasing immobility of countenance. At night, and even in bed, masks were sometimes worn to improve the complexion. Outworn day-masks were heavily creamed and pulled tightly against the face. As Michael Drayton recorded,

There be fine nightmasks
Plastered well within
To supple wrinkles
And to smooth the skin

The wearing of masks in public places soon led to an interesting compensatory process: since the female face was now so anonymously concealed, other charms could be exposed, and so followed a vogue for the revealed bosom. Popular writers of the day were outraged. Thomas

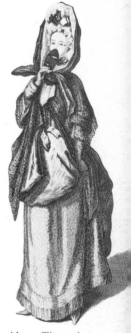

Above *The mask provided ladies of quality with new freedoms. Whilst walking abroad in the town identity passed unnoticed and in the bawdy theatre her enjoyment was unseen*

Opposite
Party mask

Travelling mask for the lady traveller of 1903

A mask for winter weather. Engraving after Winter *by Hollais*

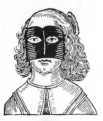

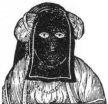

Above *Englishwomen's masks, mid-17th century*

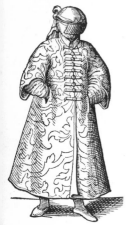

Above *A Turkish woman, late 16th century*

Centre *18th century mask*

Right *Fashionable lady motorists, 1903*

Opposite *70's veil*

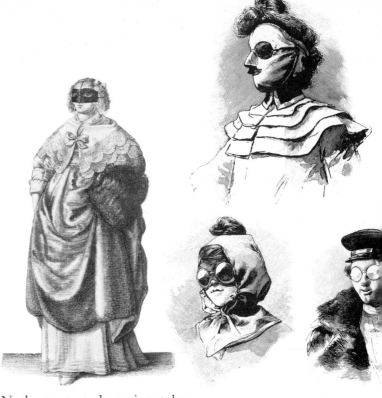

Nashe protested passionately:

> Their breastes they embuske upp on hie and their rounde roseate buds immodestly large thrust forthe and show that at their handes their is fruite to bee hoped.

The Welshman, Matthew Griffiths, spoke even more plainly:

> If your wares bee not vendible why do you open your shoppes?

The veil has enjoyed a much longer popularity than the mask, and in many more widely-separated countries. At first sight, it seems to have little more than a simple concealing function; in fact it usually succeeds in increasing attention to the face, being one of the most attractive devices for constructing a frame around it. Some unusually attractive veils were popular in Edwardian times. Together with the large hats of the day, they served to define, in a most pleasing way, an expanded visual space around the face—which was thereby made to appear all the more attractively small and precious. The veil can have the further effect of rendering the outlines of the face and the features pleasingly

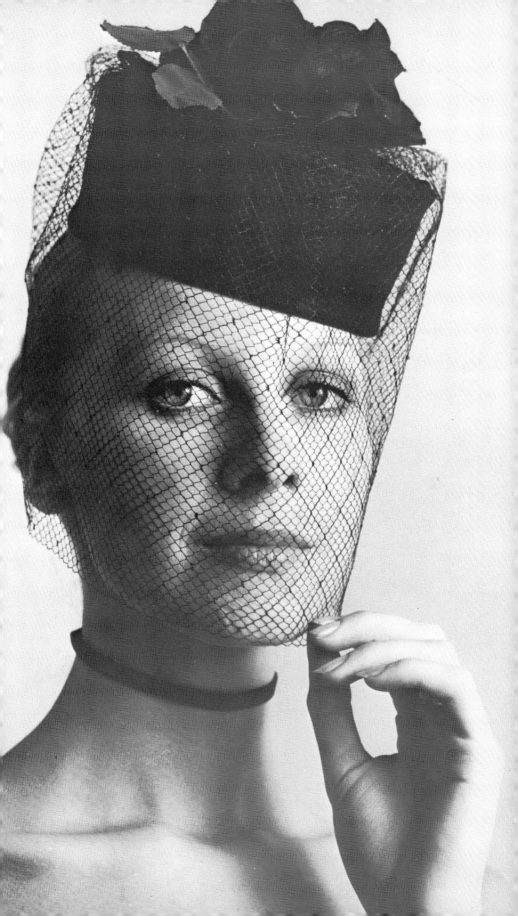

Top *Filipino fishermen believe their masks lure fish into their nets*

Bottom *A Saharan Touareg nomad from Southern Algeria in feast-day costume*

Opposite:
Top left *An Indian woman in purdah examines a film-strip at a new Education Centre in Bombay, 1952*

Top right *Tripolitanian bride, 1952*

Bottom *Housewives, Afghanistan, 1963*

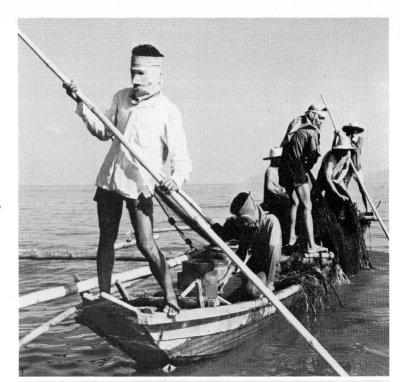

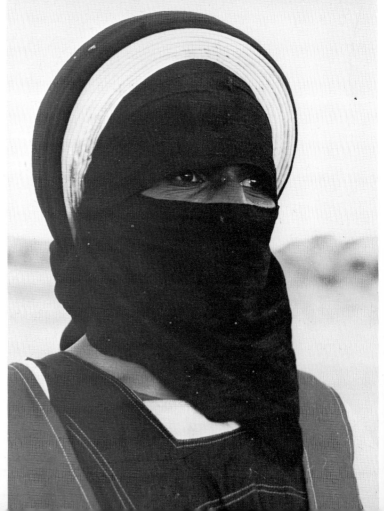

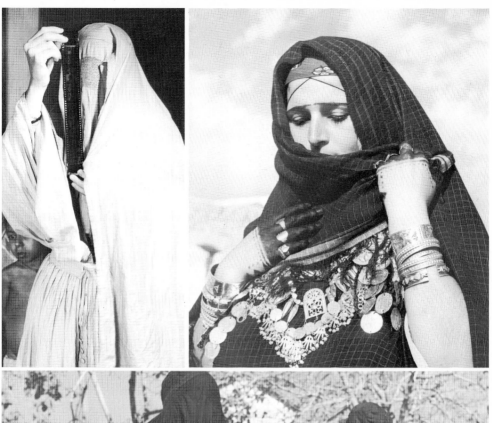

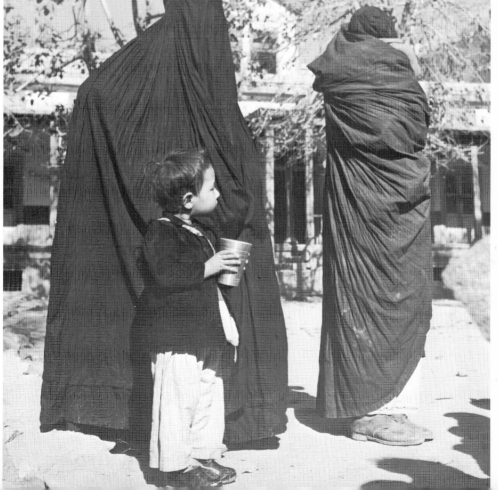

vague and indistinct, sometimes greatly enhancing the impression of beauty. Veils have the further advantage of distracting attention from natural wrinkles and lines. And the network of the veil provides a mobile variant of the face-patch or beauty-spot, highlighting by contrast the pale beauty of the skin.

The veil has firmly established itself as an international symbol of intrigue, adventure and secret assignation. In Eastern countries, girls are said to be chased by their young suitors only when they are wearing the veil. And Moslem men everywhere claim that they can readily discern whether the face beneath the veil is pretty or plain. The veil is as popular today as ever it was in Eastern and Moslem countries, where it is described variously as the Burqua, the Yashmak or the Chadri. What is its fascination? First and foremost, it is seen as a protector—not simply a physical protector, against sun and weather, but a psychological protector, which emphasises and perpetuates the attractive notion of woman's weakness and vulnerability. It has even acquired a symbolic meaning, the custom having arisen in some Eastern countries of sending the veil by messenger as a cry for help: a call which is always taken seriously and instantly obeyed. But the veil has other, more prosaic, uses. It may be a concealment, welcome alike to husband and wife, for shabbiness, drabness or ugliness. Perhaps, more important still, it secures privacy, peace and seclusion—much-valued qualities in the Moslem world. The veil symbolises, too, that other pillar of the Moslem life, the notion of equality. Wealth and nobility are accidents of birth which reflect no credit on the individual. All Moslem women are equal; all are entitled to wear the badge of equality, the veil. There have been many impassioned calls to Moslem women by politicians in recent years to give up the veil. Kemel Ataturk made such an appeal to the women of Turkey. Recently Bourgiba called again to the women of Tunisia: 'Come out from behind your veils and into the twentieth century!' But such renunciation would be too traumatic. The reasons are not hard to find. The veil is no ordinary protection; it has quite unique and, some would say, almost magical powers. In Afghanistan, even today, no child is allowed to wander out unveiled, lest wicked local spirits, known as the 'Affrits', catch sight of its face and harm it. Psychological pressures such as these are quite overwhelming and it is most unlikely that the veil will quickly disappear.

Another method of partial concealment, the fan, became widely popular in Europe at the end of the seventeenth century. Originally fans were used only by the ladies of the Court and by courtesans—but eventually, towards the end of the eighteenth century, they were adopted by most ladies of fashion. Some of these fans, painted by artists of the stature of Reynolds and Fragonard, were of great beauty. They were used everywhere—in the town and even at Church, although moralists sometimes objected, ostensibly on the grounds of the impropriety of the paintings with which many of the fans were decorated: scenes from Hogarth, for example, or the naked Graces, or Venus and Cupid, or perhaps gay life in the cities, or the Rake at sport with the women. And so 'Church Fans', painted with more sober Bible scenes, became fashionable for Holy Days. But perhaps the real objection was that fans were used for secret, silent conversations in Church. The 'language of the fan' was easy to learn—the number of struts of the partially-opened fan indicated the time for meeting—the fan pressed to the lips indicated the expectation of a kiss, the pressure of the fan across the heart, the strength of the passion. As one contemporary account put it, 'If a fan is closed across the heart then Cupid's arrow has found its mark.' Many such signals came into common use—so many in fact as to justify the publication in Spain of a *Fan Dictionary* explaining fifty or so basic phrases and their possible variations and combinations which allowed messages of great subtlety and delicacy. Many, though not all of these, were devoted to the language of love. A female needed only eye-movements and a well-handled fan to enjoy a full, even passionate, 'conversation' with her lover—and this in the most public of places and in an age of great social restraint. It is easy to see why the fan became so popular. In Spain it first came into common use at a time when rigid social and sexual prohibitions were beginning to forbid much ordinary social intercourse. Fans have even enjoyed a certain popularity with men. They were used by Iroquois Indians while

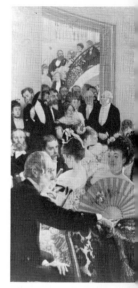

The Concert by James Tissot. (1836–1902)

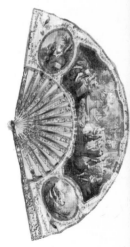

French painted fan of the 18th century

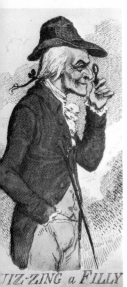

JIZ-ZING a FILLY

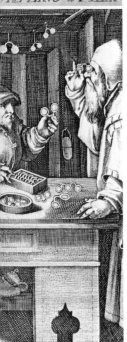

sitting around the camp fire in the evening. And like the fans of European courtiers, these Iroquois fans were often of great beauty. Some were woven from large bird feathers, like those of the wild turkey, others from carefully-plaited grasses specially chosen for their delicate fragrance. Each fan contributed its own perfume to a delightful evening ceremony which rewarded the hard business of the day. The pleasantness, and so the cohesiveness, of social life was thereby increased.

Another interesting 'defensive' device for the face became popular among fashionable men early in the nineteenth century. This was the quizzing glass, a lens held before the face with an air of great *hauteur,* which enabled one to examine one's acquaintances, or one's menu, or perhaps simply the world at large. It was a terrifying device, which intimidated shopmen and servants alike with its close, intense gaze. It provided, too, an impeccable excuse for failing to recognise an acquaintance. It was an exquisite, elegant demonstration of the languor and boredom so fashionable in Regency times. It was an ideal accessory for the dandy, with corseted figure and padded chest, rumpled hair and enamelled face. Later in the nineteenth century, a similar device for ladies, the *lorgnette,* was adopted by the fashionable and elegant, and for much the same reasons. A modern echo of this same impulse is to be found in the current vogue for the wearing of gigantic, coloured fun spectacles, which have no optical function whatsoever, but which create the flattering illusion of enormous eyes in old and young alike.

One of the strangest of all devices for concealing facial defects was the 'plumper'. This grossly uncomfortable object consisted of a pad of cotton and cork worn inside the mouth to swell the cavities left by lost teeth and shrinkage of the gums. Plumpers had the pleasing effect of filling out the cheeks and giving a flatteringly full contour to shrunken, dropped, or ageing faces. They enjoyed a surprisingly long popularity—from the time of Charles II until the end of the eighteenth century. They were not without their problems, however, as Mrs. Cowley reported in *The Belles Strategem* of 1780:

Mrs Button wears cork plumpers in each cheek and never hazards more than six words for fear of showing them.

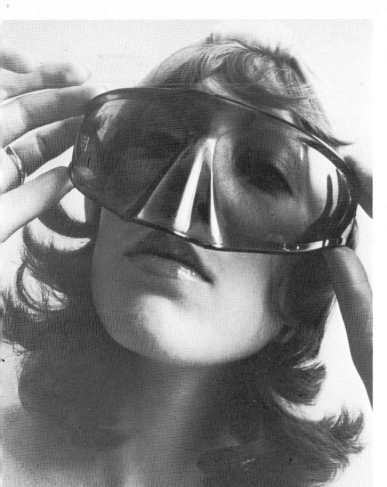

*Sun visor designed by
Oliver Goldsmith*

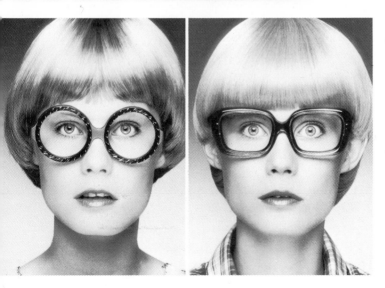

*Spectacles by Mary
Quant*

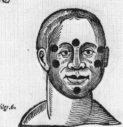

in their neather Lip downe to their Chin, and this is their Baptisme when they are made Christians,which they use in stead of water.

The *Virginian* women pounce and rase their Faces and whole Bodies with a sharp iron,which makes a stampe in curious knots, and drawes the proportions of Fowles,Fishes,or Beasts; then with painting of sundrylively colours they rub it into the stampe, which will never be taken away, because it is dried into the flesh.

Purch.Pilgr.6. lib.9.

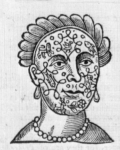

Idem Pilgr.2. lib.7.

The *Egyptian* Moores, both men and women, for love of each other, distaine their Chins into knots,and flowers of blew, made by the pricking of the skin with needles, and rubbing it over with inke and the juyce of an herb.   *what*

Barbarous Nations,are seldome known to be contented with a Face of Gods making; for they are either adding, detracting, or altering continually, having many Fucusses in readinesse for the same purpose. Sometimes they think they have too much colour, then they use Art to make them look pale and faire. Now they have too little colour,then Spanish paper,Red Leather, or other Cosmeticall Rubriques must be had. Yet for all this, it may be, the skins of their Faces do not please them; off they go with Mercury water, and so they remaine like peeld Ewes, untill their Faces have recovered a new *Epidermis*.

Our Ladies here have lately entertained a vaine Custome of spotting their Faces, out of an affectation of a Mole to setoff their beauty, such as *Venus* had, and it is well if one black patch will serve to make their Faces remarkable; for some fill their Visages full of them, varied into all manner of shapes and figures.

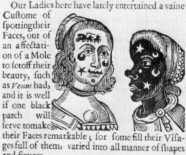

This is as odious, and as senselesse an affectation as ever was used by any barbarous Nation in the World; And I doubt our Ladies that use them are not well advised of the effect they worke: for these spots in   *Faire*

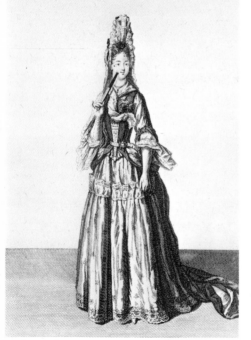

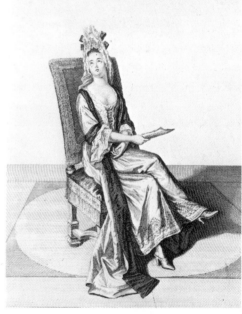

The face patch has a long and interesting history—it was popular even in the days of the Roman Empire. It became popular again at the Court of Louis XV. The fashion was by no means restricted to women: Elizabethan fops used to wear them in the shape of black crescents, stars and lozenges to improve their manly faces. They were often valued, too, by men who wore them as ostentatious concealments of honourable scars of battle, real or imaginary. The fashion persisted through several succeeding reigns. Clapthorne, writing in 1640, gave young men the following advice:

If it be a lover's part you are to act, take a black spot or two, 'twill make your face more amorous, and appear more gracious in your mistress' eyes.

Only later, according to Bulwer's *Artificial Changeling*, published in 1653, did the fashion spread to Englishwomen too:

Our ladies have lately entertained a vain custom of spotting their faces, out of an affectation of a mole, to set off their beauty, such as Venus did; and it is well if one black patch will serve to make their faces remarkable for some fill their visage full of them, varied into all manner of shapes.

He illustrated a lady's face of the time with the popular favourite, the 'Coach and horses'. Patches were often made of black taffeta or red Spanish leather. They were often placed near the mouth, and eventually came to be worn in ridiculously large sizes and patterns. Originally they had simply been 'mouches' or small love spots. In 1660, Mr. Pepys declared himself pleased with his wife's first appearance in patches:

My wife seemed pretty today, it being the first time I had given her leave to wear a black patch.

A week or two later he recorded that his wife, wearing two or three patches, 'looked far handsomer with them than the Princess Henrietta.' Sometimes, however, the effects of patches were less satisfactory: the Duchess of Newcastle was said to have presented a grotesque appearance in 1667 when she wore a black velvet cap, curls about her ears and many large patches on and around her mouth to conceal her pimples. The popularity of patches no doubt owed a great deal to their ability to conceal such blemishes of

Opposite:
Top *Two pages from Bulwer's 17th century account of the facial elaborations of the ladies of Virginia and Egypt. On the right is an English lady wearing the popular 'Coach and Horses' patch*

Bottom left *Beauty patches were worn by fashionable ladies of Paris at the end of the 17th century*

Bottom right *Patches were worn even 'en déshabillé'*

complexion and the scars of disease common enough in those days of smallpox. And of course they threw into high relief, by contrast, a pleasingly pale skin.

At Louis XV's Court, an entire 'language of patches' developed, which was eventually to become as elaborate as the 'language of the fan'. Patches on the forehead were the mark of 'majesty'; at the corner of the eye they indicated 'passion'. A patch on the centre of the cheek was 'gay', and on the nose 'saucy'. A patch on the lips was said to be an invitation to a kiss. In England, too, some quaint conventions arose: Lady Castlemaine, an authority of the times, tells for example, that 'patches cannot be worn with mourning. It is proper however to wear them at all other times—at the theatre in the afternoon, in the parks in the evening, and in the drawing room at night.' Satirists of the times poured scorn on the custom. One was driven to write in the *Spectator* 'An Invective against Black Spotted Faces'. But the fashion continued unabated, and in the time of Queen Anne, according to the *Spectator*, went on to acquire yet new significance when politically-minded ladies used their patches as party symbols. And so developed yet another language of patches: the Whigs patching on the right and the Tories on the left side of their faces—while those who were neutral decorated both cheeks. The *Spectator* of 1711 deplored 'the motives of a few fantastic coquettes who do not patch for the public good so much as for their own private advantage', but expressed its 'confidence that there are several women of honour who patch out of principle, and with an eye to the interests of their country.' One lady of the day was even reported to have stipulated in her marriage contract that whatever the opinions of her husband 'she shall be at liberty to patch on which side she pleases.' By the middle of the eighteenth century, the patches had become even larger and more numerous, so much so that a writer in 1754 expressed his concern at their concealment of essential femininity:

> It is with great sorrow that I see it in possession of that great mass of blue which borders upon the female eye . . . surely it is to be hoped the ladies will not give up that place to a plaster, which the brightest jewel in the universe would want lustre to supply.

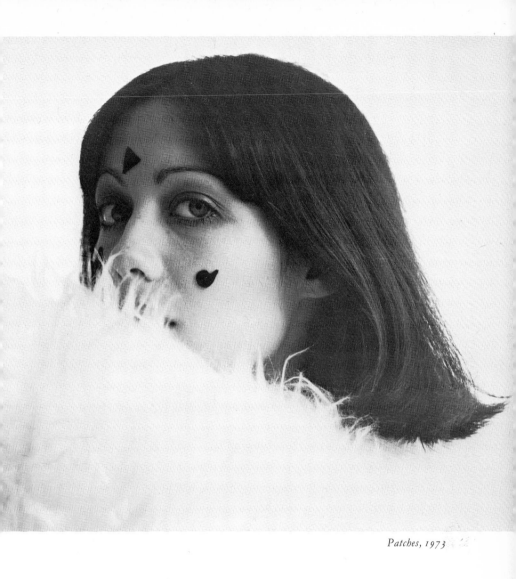

Patches, 1973

7 Changing the structure

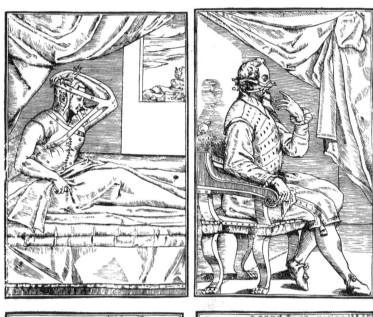

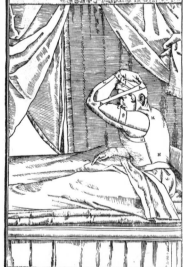

Opposite *These illustrations from Tagliacozzi's textbook show the remarkable sophistication of techniques in cosmetic surgery even as long ago as the 16th century*

There is nothing new about cosmetic surgery; it was being practised at least a thousand years ago in India. And during the Middle Ages, the anatomists Vesalius, Fallopius and Ambroise Paré all wrote warning surgeons about its dangers and difficulties. The first printed work on the subject, Tagliacozzi's *De Chirurgia Curtorum,* published in 1597, contains twenty-two detailed woodcuts illustrating facial operations in progress. Tagliacozzi himself achieved much success during his lifetime, and his services were eagerly sought. But this did not save him from being posthumously denounced as a sorcerer. The mediaeval church was opposed to such interference with God's work, and Tagliacozzi's body was exhumed and re-interred in unhallowed ground. One of his original operative procedures is still in use today and still bears his name. The *Madras Gazette* of 1793 gave a detailed account of an operation undertaken to replace a nose lost in a duel. The method used, described as 'always successful', was to bring down a flap of tissue from the forehead. This again is a procedure still used today. An even more delicate operation was reported by Carl von Graefe in 1809 for the repair of the damaged eyelid of a young girl. He used the same basic method— bending back a flap of tissue—but in this case upwards from the cheek. In *The Gentleman's Magazine* of 1814, there is another detailed account of a successful facial repair.

It was long ago discovered that facial tissue is in many ways ideal for surgery, being so well supplied with blood vessels; artificial flaps show little tendency to necrose or die, as they might well be expected to do. It was little more than a century ago, however, that the really important discovery was made by Reverdin that even a completely detached flap of tissue and skin could live and grow satis- factorily in a quite different area of the same person's body, provided the new area had been suitably prepared for it. This discovery was a quite revolutionary one, and opened up a whole range of new possibilities in plastic surgery. Several new techniques were described in 1928 by Jacques Joseph in his *Nasenplastik und sonstige Gesichtsplastik.* As well as pioneering these new techniques Joseph invented many of the special tools, such as elevators and saws, which are now in widespread use for reducing the size of nasal cartilage and bone.

The greatest triumphs of cosmetic surgery are in the repair of the disfigurements suffered in road accidents and warfare. It is in these cases particularly that there can be disastrous psychological, as well as physical damage. Quite profound changes in the whole picture of the self often seem to be brought about by such facial mutilations; destruction of the face seems all too frequently to bring about destruction of the whole personality. In cases such as these, painstaking rebuilding of the face and intensive psychological care can bring enormous happiness, given time and generous patience. Concurrently with the physical repair comes a new access of life and hope: the patient gradually begins to feel that he is fit once again to rejoin the human race. Fine work is done, too, by plastic surgeons in the reconstruction of malformations, such as the hare-lip, caused by accidents of genetics. Until recently people born with such conditions often suffered heartbreaking feelings of ugliness and shame. But techniques have now been perfected, like those of König and Mirault, which almost invisibly knit together the loose edges of the cleft—an operation which is best undertaken in babyhood, before any psychological harm has been done. Many other genetic disfigurements, like birthmarks and naevi ('port-wine stains'), and malformations such as the unearned saddle-nose of congenital syphilis, all nowadays respond to the surgeon's knife. But a great deal of happiness is achieved also by the correction of faults far less serious than these: humped noses, receding chins and 'bat ears' can all now be altered by routine surgical procedures. Prominent ears can easily be flattened, as the surgeon Morestin demonstrated more than fifty years ago. This is a fairly widespread condition, caused either by over-development of the concha or by under-development of the antihelix; contrary to popular belief, it has nothing whatsoever to do with the carelessness of mothers so often blamed in the past for 'allowing their children to sleep on a folded ear.' The operation consists simply of the removal of a crescent of skin from just behind the ear and a similar crescent from the pinna, or ear flap, and then stitching together. Again, it is possible to reduce the overall size of unduly large ears, and even to

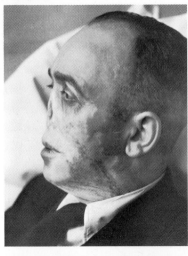
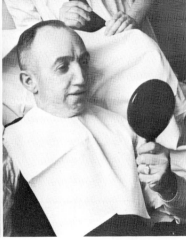

One of the earliest cosmetic surgery operations undertaken under the National Health Service: repair of a damaged nose in the early 1940s

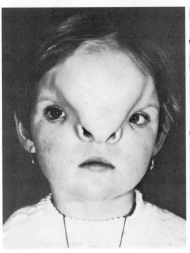
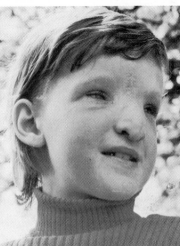

Surgical correction of Hypertelorism (Grieg's disease) involving removal of a section of the nose and the forehead

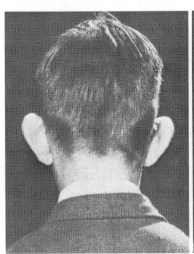
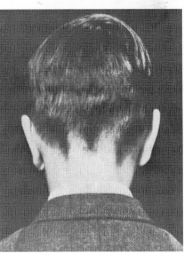

The flattening of outstanding ears

construct ears for those people unfortunate enough to be born without them. These operations can generate much happiness, perhaps even more for men than for women, who at least have the option of concealing their ears behind their hair.

Moralists sometimes object to such 'interference with nature'. Sometimes, too, there may be good psychological grounds for discouraging the unrealistic pursuit of youth which sometimes prompts requests for facial surgery. Yet it must be pointed out that much psychological harm may be done by withholding treatment from a sensitive child who worries unnecessarily about his 'bat ears' or from the young woman who cannot face men because of a nose she feels to be ugly. Simple operations can bring them both much happiness. Brown and McDowall, the authors of the standard text, *Plastic Surgery of the Nose*, have little patience with those who object on moral grounds: they insist that 'the wish of the individual patient is the primary consideration. The patient's desire for the correction of a deformity is the main reason for undertaking a rhinoplastic procedure.'

Even relatively minor imperfections of the skin can cause much distress. Adolescents in particular are highly sensitive about their skin; they may even become emotionally withdrawn simply because they feel it to be disfigured by acne. This common condition is produced by nothing more than the clogging of sebaceous glands, which is followed by the production of comedones, or blackheads, behind which bacteria multiply producing pustules. Administration of hormones may sometimes bring about some improvement, in girls especially, though the condition is often resistant to medical treatment. If neglected, it may sometimes lead to pitting of the face and permanent loss of elasticity in the skin. One method of treatment for acne was mentioned as long ago as 1500 BC in the *Papyrus Ebers*. It consisted of the use of an abrasive made from alabaster and grain. Before the First World War, E. Kromayer advocated a similar treatment involving even harsher abrasion—with dental burrs and rasps. More recently, at least one surgeon has advocated the use of an electrically powered wire brush. The skin is evidently much tougher than we think.

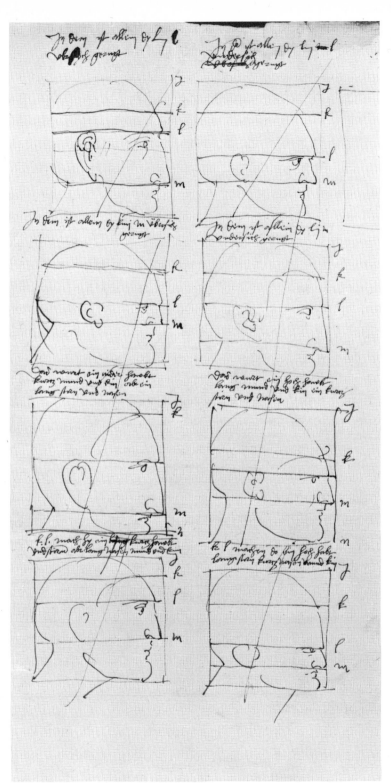

Dürer, like Leonardo,
believed that the nose
determined the whole
character of the face.
This page from one of
Dürer's notebooks
shows his preoccupation
with nasal proportions

Left *A photograph
taken in March, 1965,
of singer Tom Jones*

Right *Tom Jones on
location in 1972 during
the making of his T.V.
programme:* The
Special London
Bridge Special

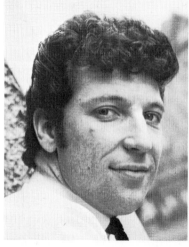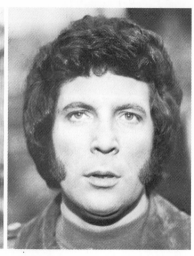

Middle & bottom:
*Before and after nasal
surgery. Patients of
Dr. Bourguet of the
French Academy of
Medicine, 1924*

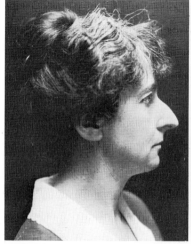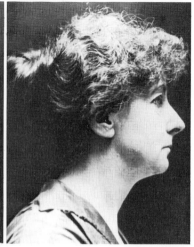

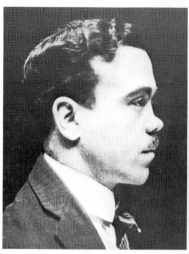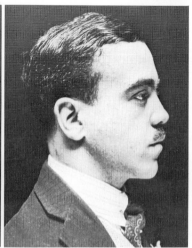

By far the greater proportion of the cosmetic surgeon's work is concerned with rhinoplasty, the alteration of the shape of the nose. This is hardly surprising, since, of all the features, it is the nose which most profoundly affects facial appearance. Leonardo da Vinci was convinced that the nose set the whole character of a face. Dürer, too, demonstrated in his drawings the remarkable transformations which could be produced by quite minor alterations in its length. The physiognomist Lavater expressed the view that the whole attractiveness of the face depended crucially on the nose. Schopenhauer cynically observed that 'the fate of so many women depends on a slight up or down curve of their nose.' Bertillon, the criminologist, was so convinced that the nose was the key to the individuality of the face that he advocated careful measurement of the nose in the compilation of criminal records. Even changes of apparent identity can be brought about by quite small alterations to the nose—as is well known by war-criminals, spies and others anxious to escape recognition. International stars and celebrities evidently set great store by it too. Tom Jones, Cilla Black, Vince Hill and Millicent Martin, among others, have all thought it well worth while to improve on nature.

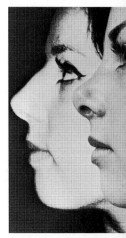

Much happiness can be generated by cosmetic surgery: a nose before and after

One of the great advantages of nasal surgery is that it can almost always be undertaken from within the nostrils, so that it leaves no unsightly scars. A humped-nose may be reduced, for example, by the quite painless removal of cartilage from inside the nose, with a small bayonet saw. Twisted noses, too, can be straightened quite easily from inside the nose by slight removals of bone and re-positioning of tissue. Much of the hard structure of the nose happens to consist of cartilage and is consequently much easier to modify than bone. Ugly, oversized noses are often caused by excessive size of the lower lateral cartilage, which is relatively easy to remove after a temporary separation has been made of the superficial skinny layers from the cartilage itself. Alterations of nasal shape can sometimes be achieved even more readily by simple modifications to the soft tissues. Noses which are too large can easily be improved by having soft flesh removed from the tip or from the tissues overlying the septum. A particularly successful example of this is the operation for the removal of flesh and hypertrophied lateral tissue from the unsightly 'potato nose'. This, incidentally, is one of the few nasal operations requiring incisions to be made from the outside; consequently it leaves small scars. The overall improvement is usually so great, however, that there are few complaints. Small scars are sometimes left, too, by operations for reducing the width or the size of the nostrils—but these can usually be hidden in the *rugae* or natural folds of the cheeks. Nostrils which are too small are usually caused by an excess of thick cartilage which can easily be removed. Again, tipped-up noses can be improved by trimming of cartilage. Noses can also be increased in size: there are now available routine techniques for the insertion of ivory or bone implants to build up nasal bones or areas of cartilage which are too small. This is the method usually employed to correct the sunken bridge of the 'saddle nose' of congenital syphilis.

Implants are often used, too, for improving the shape of a receding chin. Here a very carefully shaped piece of preserved human bone, or bovine cartilage, or even polythene, is introduced through a small lateral incision below the chin. Alternatively the insert may be introduced through the floor of the mouth. Occasionally bone from the patient's own iliac bone is used, or sometimes cartilage from his ribs. Operations for correcting the 'lantern jaw' are also available. Sometimes, however, altering the chin is not

'Facial rejuvenation'

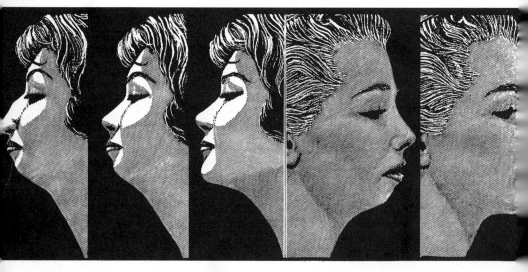

enough. According to the British plastic surgeon Gardiner, people seeking an operation for a receding chin often require rhinoplasty as well—and, as he explains in his book *Faces, Figures and Feelings*, it becomes a matter of some delicacy to explain to them that 'improvement' of the jaw line might actually worsen their appearance if the nose also were not altered at the same time. Even alterations to the size of the mouth are now regarded by surgeons as routine operative procedures. Where the mouth is too large, a V-shaped piece of flesh may be removed from the centre line and the edges then rejoined in several stages. Where the mouth is too small an incision can be made in the centre and skin and flesh grafted between the exposed edges. Operations are also frequently undertaken on the lips themselves—and in some cases this refashioning may constitute an extremely powerful aid to mental well-being. Advances in procedure are constantly being made; new techniques are now available, such as the so-called 'Z-plasty' operation for removing and repairing the scar and reducing the distortion and tension which sometimes persist from hare-lip repairs undertaken in infancy. Undue prominence or 'eversion' of the lips is now amenable to alteration. A new technique is also gaining favour for removing the fine lines which so often tend to develop above the mouth; this consists of the injection of silicone substances into the flesh above the upper lips.

The fine, 'crows feet' lines beside the eyes—and the hoods

Removal of pouches in lower eyelids

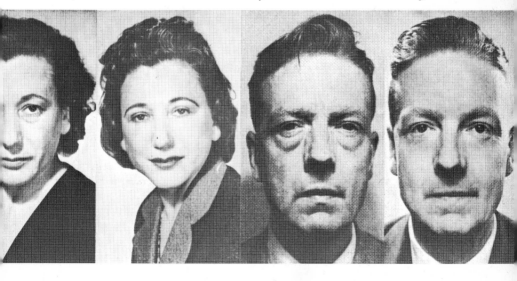

or bags which develop above and below the eyes can now be reduced by relatively simple operations. Baggy eyes are often produced by the rupturing of the fat around the eyes due to the weakness of the *orbicularis* muscles. In the corrective operation an incision is made in this muscle to permit the fat to ooze out and to be cut away. A marked change in appearance may result. Even more dramatic changes are brought about by the removal of the fat in the epicanthic folds over the upper lids, the presence of which can so often produce an unpleasant 'menacing' aspect. After the removal of this fat a certain amount of the skin of the eyelids is also removed to achieve a smooth effect—only a small amount, however, if proper mobility of the lids is to be preserved. Operations of this kind have been much in demand by television actors, since the 'hooded-eye' is one which no amount of make-up can conceal—and the television close-up is particularly searching. The eyebrows can be lifted, and the effects may be profound since, as we shall see in a later chapter, the separation of eye and eyebrow is one of the most powerful single influences on facial appearance. The popular 'forehead lift' operation for removal of 'worry lines' often has the added effect, usually felt to be an advantage, of lifting the brows. The operation consists simply of making an incision in the scalp one and a half inches behind the hairline from ear to ear, separating carefully the skin from the underlying tissue, removing some of the skin, and restitching. The resultant scar is hidden behind the hairline. But this operation is best restricted to women, since it is important that the hairline should not subsequently recede. Another simple operation, sometimes described as an 'office procedure' (one which can be undertaken in the surgeon's office) is for the removal of 'glabellar wrinkles', which produce a knot of lines between the eyebrows. A half-inch cut is made at the nasal end of the eyebrows, the skin is undermined and the fibres of the *corrugator supercilii* muscles are severed from the undersurface of the skin. In cases where the wrinkles are very pronounced, fat or some other substance is sometimes also introduced below the skin.

Apart from nose operations, the most frequent requests to the cosmetic surgeon are for face-lift and facial rejuvenation ('rhitidoplasty' and 'meloplasty'). Sagging cheeks are corrected by two small, well-chosen cuts and by removal of skin at the hair-line over the ears. If performed skilfully, this kind of operation can also correct a drooping jowl and perhaps even a double chin. More often, however, double chins are reduced by a 'chin lift', which involves removal of fat through an elliptical incision. A chin-lift should, according to Gardiner, always be supplemented by a face-lift. The face-lift itself is painless and requires the patient to remain in bandages for no more than five days. The essence of the method is to remove the skin from certain areas so that the remaining skin fits more smoothly over the under-lying fat and muscle. This undermining and detachment of skin requires great skill and delicacy of touch. Its effects are said to last up to ten years, and even then there is no reason why the operation should not be repeated. Contrary to popular belief, the tendency towards sagging of the face is not increased by face-lifting.

Though, like appendectomy, these operations are now considered routine surgery, they are not without risk and it goes without saying that they should be undertaken only by the most competent and experienced surgeons and in the best possible conditions. Though the large blood-supply naturally provided to facial tissue makes recovery rapid, there can be surgical difficulties, such as copious bleeding: these are not techniques for amateurs. Such is the popularity of these procedures, however, that special clinics have begun to appear in Paris and other large cities which offer 'mini-face-lifts' and similar 'while-you-wait' procedures for producing tucks in the skin—and these are enjoying great popularity. About ten percent of their clients are said to be male. But the results of such abbreviated methods are usually much less satisfactory than those of the more orthodox procedures, and, according to Gardiner, may even produce facial distortions. The financial cost of facial surgery may be considerable. A face-lift may cost about £500 (approximately $1,200), the removal of bags below the eyes or the lifting of eyebrows £300. Smoothing a forehead or straightening a hump-nose might cost £300.

It is now recognised that cosmetic surgery is not without dangers of a quite different kind: there may be psychological difficulties. The patient may not always be pleased with the results—and he never has the option of going back. In North Carolina not very long ago, one disgruntled patient shot the surgeon who had operated on him. And the Mayo clinic recently warned surgeons, 'Considerable patience may be needed to make these people understand that the plastic surgeon cannot make a silk purse out of a sow's ear.' But there may be more subtle psychological difficulties. Paul Schilder has warned of the dangers of 'personality regression' which might follow operations on the face: the patient might become immature and childlike. It is now known that facial blemishes are sometimes used by patients as a 'hook' on which to hang all their feelings of inadequacy. Strange beliefs about facial blemishes sometimes develop; adolescents for example, often confess to the feeling that their masturbation shows in their face, causing their blemishes to appear. In consequence they ask for the blemishes to be removed, to reduce their feelings of guilt. Schilder has suggested that the face is in fact one of the most important areas of the body in the development of a sense of personal identity. The face, he says, is often felt to *be* the self, and so in the mind's illogical way, a fine new beautiful face is believed automatically to bestow a fine and new, beautiful character. Neurotic individuals in particular often feel that their inadequacies are actually *caused* by their imperfect face, and that modification of their face will automatically rectify their personality difficulties. Cosmetic surgeons themselves declare that the best results do not follow surgery sought in this way for the solution of neurotic problems. Those who profit most are the patients who have accidental or genetic disfigurement or who seek repair for frankly cosmetic reasons. Nonetheless, neurotic individuals are often elated for a while after their operation; they usually relapse however into further and even deeper depression when they realise that life has not, after all, been miraculously changed. Such patients are sometimes depersonalised following their operation: they may feel that their face 'doesn't look right' or that it 'doesn't belong to me'. Sometimes, too, they become suspicious of their doctors and may even become difficult to treat.

The reasons given for seeking treatment are many. It

sometimes happens, for example, that patients declare that their marriage depends on the perpetuation of their cherubic beauty. If this is the case then their married life is surely in need of more than help from surgeons. Society itself, and particularly perhaps the mass media, cannot be considered blameless here: they promote and perpetuate a widespread striving for impossibly high standards of personal physical beauty. Again, patients sometimes plead that professional or vocational demands make facial surgery imperative. In certain cases this may very well be so, but the possibility should also be recognised that the patient might be deluding himself with a thinly-veiled rationalisation of an unrealistic impulse to return to one of his earlier 'seven ages'. If it is contentment which is being sought, then there must also be self-acceptance. For many people, cosmetic surgery may very well help to achieve this. For others, however, more permanently discontented, it will do little. The crucial issue is not 'self-improvement' but 'self acceptance', without which there can be little happiness.

Beauty

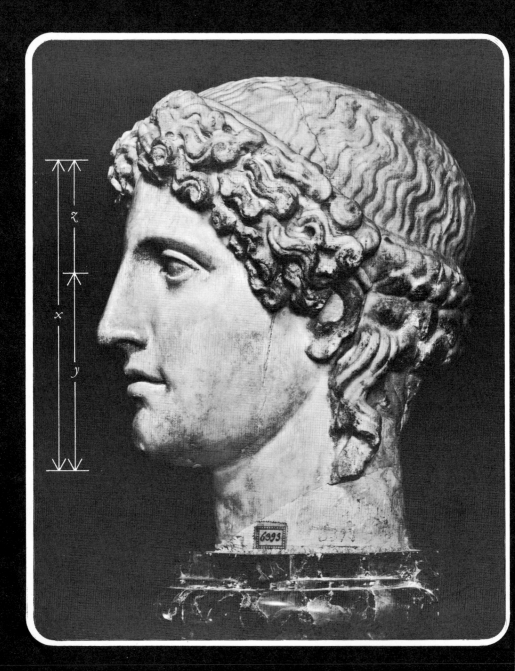

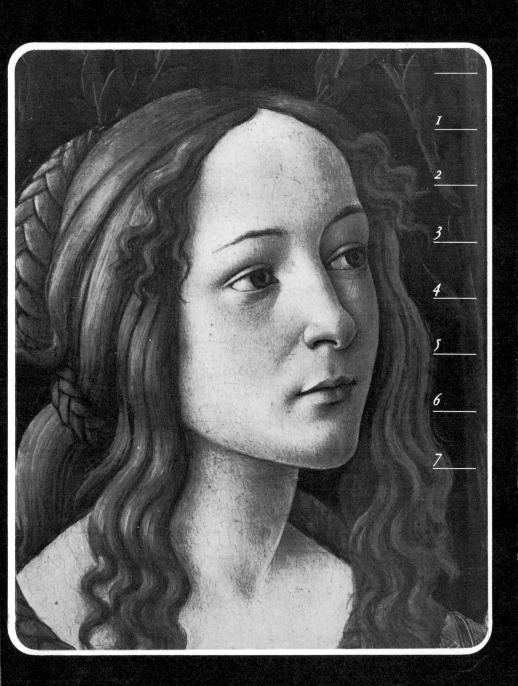

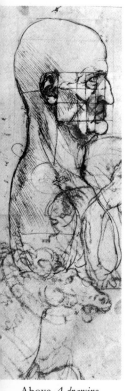

Above *A drawing from one of Leonardo da Vinci's notebooks shows his preoccupation with facial proportions*

For the ancient Greeks the idea of beauty seemed easy to define: it was a question of harmony, balance and above all of *proportion*. As Plato explained, its essence lay in the 'golden section', a special way of subdividing an object so that the smaller part is to the greater as the greater is to the whole. This formula, as our illustration shows, implied that all beautiful things have some kind of break or division about one third of the way along their length. In the 'perfect' face, therefore, the brow would be one third of the way down from the hairline and the mouth one third of the way up from the point of the chin. Again, the width of the face would be two-thirds of its height.

Mediaeval artists were more impressed by the magical number seven: they believed that the perfect face was neatly divisible not so much into thirds as into sevenths. The hair occupied the top seventh. The forehead extended over the next two sevenths, and the nose over another two sevenths. A further seventh was occupied by the space between nose and mouth and the final seventh from mouth to chin. Another rule, long popular with artists, was that the eyes should each occupy one fifth of the width of the face and that there should be the width of one eye between the eyes. Yet another decreed that the width of the face should be twice the length of the nose.

It is curious how long this search for the 'mathematical secrets' of beauty has persisted. Even as late as the eighteenth century, men of the stature of Sir Joshua Reynolds and Chevreul were still hunting for the perfect arithmetical formula—in the sure conviction that beauty was simply a matter of physical proportions. Even Hogarth was convinced there was some simple overriding principle. He believed he had found it in 'the wavy line of beauty'. He declared that 'the greatest, indeed the indispensable element of all beautiful things is the smooth serpentine line'—the soft, flowing contour such as we see in a woman's shoulder and neckline, or in the gentle curve from the brow to the tip of her nose.

Many observers have been impressed, like the Greeks, with the importance of balance and symmetry. The perfectly beautiful face was one which had perfect symmetry. Yet symmetry, as Francis Bacon long ago realised, can be

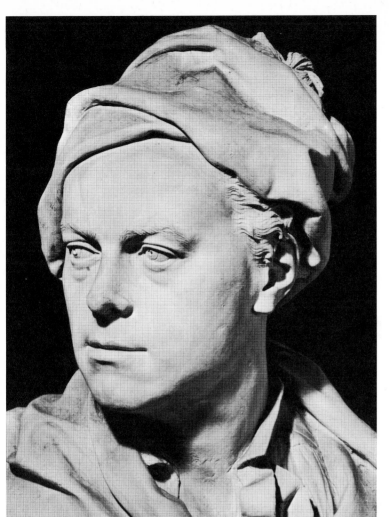

Hogarth. Portrait bust by Roubillac

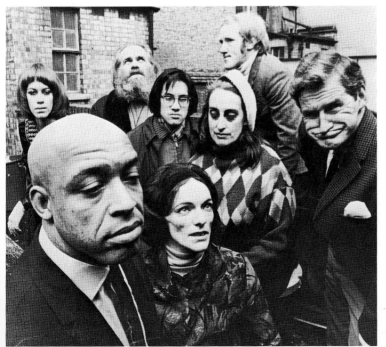

Self-confessed ugliness: volunteers for a new model agency, 'The Uglies'. But ugliness is no easier to define than beauty

exceedingly boring. 'There is no excellent beauty,' he declared, 'which hath not some strangeness in the proportion.'

Others, of more philosophical disposition, have searched for more abstract principles to explain beauty. Kant believed he had at last found the secret in 'simplicity'. Beautiful things, he said, are those which are 'easy to know', easy to comprehend. Modern psychologists, especially those of the Gestalt school, have found much in their research to support this view. Simple shapes, they have discovered, are almost invariably more pleasing to behold than more complex forms. And the Gestalt psychologists have enunciated yet another important principle: our perceptions and judgements of the world and of people are determined not so much by the detail of what we see as by the whole *pattern* of our experience at a particular moment. The beauty of a face is not so much a matter of its detail—of skin or nose or eye—as of the whole configuration created by a hundred such details interacting and affecting one another and in turn being acted upon by the surroundings, by the context and by the whole perceptual framework in which the face is enclosed at the moment. Beauty, then, is a *total* experience.

Nonetheless, most accounts of female beauty have tended to concentrate on its detail—perhaps for the good reason that patterns, configurations and contexts are extremely difficult to represent in words. Many commentators have applauded smooth, unblemished, lively complexions, and gently curved, unbroken planes and surfaces in the face. Large eyes, and eyes which are 'liquid', 'deep' or 'dreamy', 'contemplative' or 'reposed', seem always to have captured the hearts of admirers. It is interesting to discover just how constant and unchanging men's preferences have been over the centuries. Consider Curry's account of the mediaeval ideal:

> . . . blonde, golden hair, like gold wire, eyes sparkling bright and light blue, cheeks lily white or rose pink, teeth white, evenly set, arms long, snow white hands, white, long slender fingers, waist small and willowy, skin everywhere dazzling white and as silk in softness.

This, in almost every detail, echoes the modern American

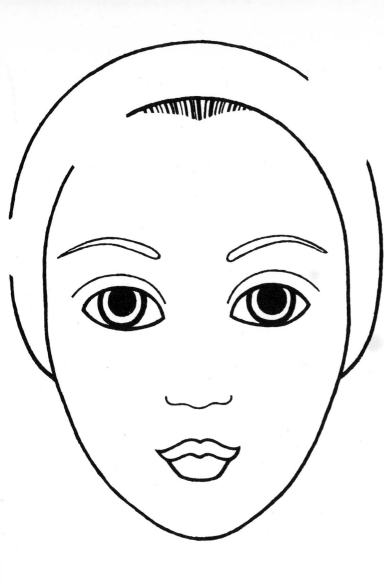

Beauty

Ancient and modern ideals of female beauty have a great deal in common

Hair
Blonde golden hair like gold wire M
Straight not crinkly B
Glossy, healthy S
Facial outline
Face oval B
Face small and round M
Eyebrows
Fine or entirely removed M *Fine* B
Fine, shapely S
Nose
Small M
Straight and diamond-shaped B
Small and slim S
Mouth
Sweet, gracious, small, soft, red or ruddy M
Soft S *Lips fine* B
Forehead
Smooth S
Eyes
Sparkling bright, light blue M
Large and blue B
Large, widely spaced, clear, bright S
Ears
Small M
Neither protruding nor large B *Small* S
Complexion
Lily-white or rose pink soft as silk M
Clear B *Smooth, clear* S

M = *Mediaeval ideal (according to Curry)*
B = *Modern American ideal (according to Brislin)*
S = *Modern Student opinion (according to Liggett)*

Brislin's 'Beauty-score' system *for both sexes*

		male	both	female	score male	female
Hair	straight		4			
	wavy		3			3
	wiry		2			
	crinkly		1			
Eyebrows	bushy	2		1		
	fine	1		2		
Eyes	small		2			
	large		3			3
	protruding		1			
	blue		2			2
	other colours		1			
Eyelashes	notably long		2			
	not long		1			1
Nose	straight *in profile*		4			4
	upturned		3			
	droopy	1		2		
	roman	2		1		
	straight *front view*		2			
	blobby *large tip*		1			
	diamond-shaped		3			
Complexion	clear		4			4
	freckled	1		2		
	marked		1			
Shape of face	oval		3			
	round	1		2		2
	squarish	2		1		
Ears	protruding		1			
	small lobes		2			2
	neither		5			
Mouth	notably wide or narrow		0			0
	fine lips		1			
	neither		3			
	Add total from *Overall proportions*					
						21

Brislin's beauty scoring method based on a survey he made in North America. Adapted from Brislin, 1962

Additional score for Overall proportions: *Start with 20 points. Deduct 5 points if brow-height is not greater than chin-height. Deduct 5 points if twice cheek-width (viewed from front) is greater than mouth-width. Add to 'features' score. Maximum possible Beauty Score= 55 points*

ideal: a recent American survey by Cuber provided almost word for word, the same prescription. In Britain, too, patterns of preference seem similar as the author found in a survey of student opinion. A beautiful female face should, according to the majority view, have large, widely-spaced, soft eyes with long lashes. The nose should be small and slim, the skin clear, pale and smooth and the cheek bones high. The mouth should be medium-sized or small, and soft, with gentle lips which are not too thick. Another recent survey, by the American psychologist Brislin, found that people were in such agreement about the constituents of beauty that it was possible to compute a 'beauty score' for every face. To score best of all on Brislin's scale, the face (male or female) had to be oval in shape, the complexion clear, the eyes large, preferably blue, and the lashes long; the nose straight and 'diamond-shaped' (when viewed from the front), the mouth of moderate size (neither wide nor narrow). The ears had neither to protrude nor to have small lobes. To score well, men needed bushy eyebrows; women had to have brows which were fine. A roman nose scored well for a man but not so well for a woman. For males a square face scored better than a round face (though not as well as an oval face). Brislin's 'beauty score' took into account not only the separate features of the face, but also the overall proportions. The proportion of the central area occupied by nose, mouth and eyes to the total facial area, for example, was important. The forehead-height had to be greater than the chin-height, and the width of the cheeks seen from the front had not to be greater than the width of the mouth.

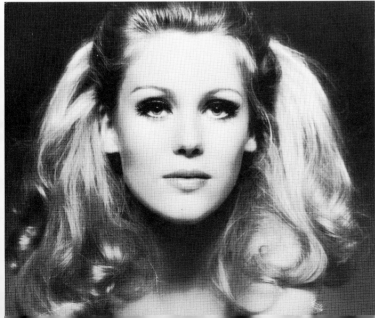

A Helena Rubinstein ideal of the seventies

A 1972 survey by the author of 100 students' opinions showed that males and females had rather different ideas about masculinity and femininity

Features are ranked according to the number of times they were mentioned in response to the questions:

What are the most important characteristics of a feminine face?	What are the most important characteristics of a masculine face?
1 Eyes large and wide apart	1 Firm jaw and wide chin
2 Smooth skin	2 Large or 'strong' mouth
3 Full mouth, soft lips	3 Clear eyes
4 Small nose	4 Facial hair and stubbly skin
5 Clear complexion	5 Large or strong nose
6 Delicate features	6 Hair grooming and style
7 Rounded cheekbones	
8 Small chin	
9 Small ears	

NB When the 50 males and the 50 females were considered separately: on 'femininity' the females were found to attach more importance to smooth skin, clear complexion, and large eyes than did the males; whereas the males attached more importance to delicate features and hair than did the females.

On 'masculinity' the females attached more importance to firm jaw, strong mouth, facial hair and stubbly skin than did males. The males, on the other hand, attached more importance to hair length and style than did the females.

Opposite *Marilyn Monroe*

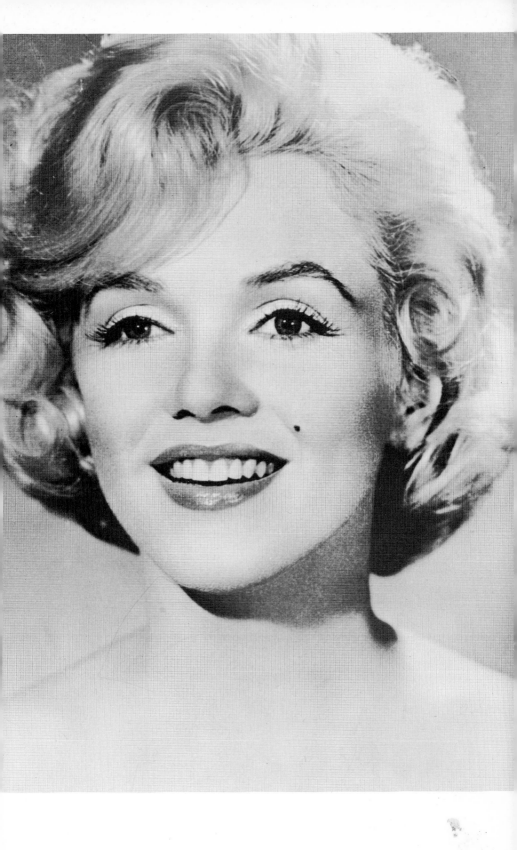

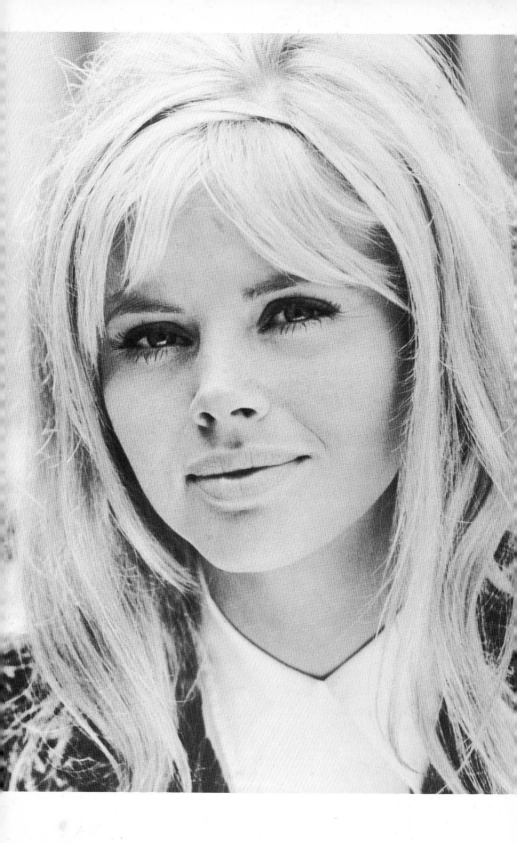

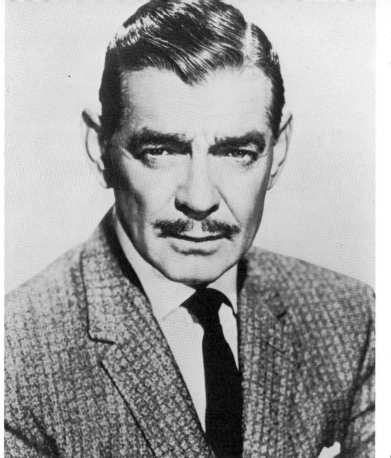

Clark Gable

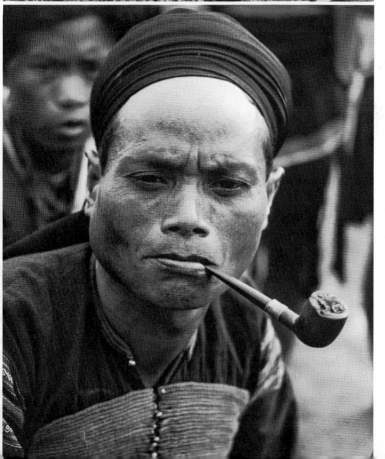

*Man of the Moi people
of Vietnam*

But surely these physical factors are only part of the story. It is the whole *pattern* of experience at a particular moment that we feel to be beautiful or unbeautiful. This pattern is composed not merely of visual sensations but also of impressions and memories from within ourselves. Most of all perhaps it stems from a whole collection of interpretations and inferences about the personality, the values, and the standards of the person we believe to exist *behind* the face. In short, our experience of beauty depends upon a whole collection of complex mental processes—not just on simple visual sensations.

Several different theories have been proposed to account for the mental processes underlying our experience of beauty. Perhaps the most famous is that which has been suggested by psychoanalytic writers who declare that our experience of beauty has its true origins in the unconscious mind, the part of the mind which contains a great 'libidinal' force striving for life or love. This 'life force', in Freud's view, is often unable to find direct satisfaction because of the practical realities of life in our sexually restrictive society. When the sexual aim is denied direct release it can still gain satisfaction in an indirect, 'sublimated' form in the experience of, or the creation of, things of beauty. The experience of beauty, according to this view, arises essentially from feelings of sensual excitement, which become transformed into *aesthetic* feelings when the primary sexual aim is, for any reason, wholly or partially inhibited. The American sociologist Frumkin takes a somewhat similar view. Human beauty is judged by the 'function' or 'potential function' of what is seen. A female is judged beautiful or not according to her 'sexual aptitude'. She is beautiful 'not only because of the symmetry or proportions or features of her form but also because of the potential sexual functions suggested by this form.' This kind of theory explains at least the almost universal valuation of youth and health as qualities which are in themselves beautiful; both youth and health tend to exaggerate the differences between the sexes and to heighten the performances in which the sexes respectively excel—strength and vigour in the male and child-bearing in the female. Any physical features felt to be conducive to these will naturally appear beautiful to the opposite sex. It is for reasons like this, according to Havelock Ellis, that a pregnant woman is often thought to be especially beautiful. As we have seen in earlier chapters, it has often been the objective of cosmetic and other elaborations of the face and its surroundings to exaggerate the naturally-occurring differences between male and female. Where such devices have been successful in this purpose they have usually been accounted 'beautiful'. But the idea that sexual attractiveness and beauty are equivalent has been attacked from many sides, notably by Simone de Beauvoir. She believes that the experience of 'beauty' is much more than mere sensual feelings arising from sexual desire. Schopenhauer went a good deal further: beauty had nothing whatsoever to do with sex:

> It is only the man whose intellect is clouded by the sexual impulse that could give the name of the *fair sex* to that undersized, narrow-shouldered, broad-hipped and short-legged race; for the whole so-called 'beauty' of the sex is bound up with this sexual impulse. Instead of calling them beautiful there would be more warrant for describing women as the 'unaesthetic sex'.

Beauty, for Schopenhauer, was a subtle, abstract and complex intellectual experience, yet one which was of the highest possible importance to us all because the contemplation of true beauty was our sole salvation from 'the tyranny of the passions'.

Many psychologists would agree that the experience of beauty involves a great deal more than sexual feelings. People are seen to be beautiful because of their mind and outlook, their character, and, particularly perhaps, their capacity for affection. Beauty is a quality of the whole person—not just his or her physical attributes. There is a strong association in the mind between virtue and beauty. This belief is reflected in folklore and literature, where heroines have always been beautiful, and villains ugly. And heroines' thoughts and deeds have been beautiful too. From his research at Johns Hopkins University, Dr. H. Huber has found that people do sincerely believe that those with the pleasantest personalities are indeed the more beautiful. There might well be a causal link, he suggested—perhaps beauty of personality actually *enhanced* facial beauty:

Thinking and feeling along noble lines are reflected in the harmonious play of the mimetic musculature. Disturbing associated movements are thereby eliminated and facial expressions may thus attain admirable beauty.

Two thousand years previously, Sappho had had very much the same idea: 'What is beautiful is good,' she declared, 'and who is good will soon be beautiful.'

Modern research has uncovered some unexpected sources for our experience of beauty. Nostalgia, for example, seems to count for a good deal; memories of 'significant persons' in our past carry over into our present attitudes and may play an overwhelming part in determining what sorts of persons we now judge to be rewarding, pleasant and beautiful. Memories of mothers, fathers and early loves all seem to play a crucial part; we often display our desire to perpetuate them in the faces we gather around us, and sometimes, too, in the faces of those we marry. Happy and unhappy experiences in our formative years leave indelible marks on our preferences. The faces of those we loved in childhood—those who were warm and comforting—live on in our mind. And memories of the faces of those we feared, hated or despised may equally affect our present judgements of beauty.

Much depends, too, on wider influences on our life— even the decorative objects, paintings and pictures which we have grown accustomed to seeing around us. Madge Garland believes that our conceptions of beauty spring from art. It is the artists, she insists, who create our standards. André Gide shares this view: it is the artists who create and define the standards of beauty which later generations subsequently endorse. There is no aspect of our everyday experience which is not modified by art. 'Even sunsets,' he said, 'have never been the same since Turner!' Film and television, too, are, without question, important shapers of our taste, especially so since the feeling still lingers on, however unconsciously, that what we see on the screen is somehow official and 'approved'. Again, our ideas of attractiveness and beauty depend to a surprising degree on familiarity, on what has been customary in our particular environment. The anthropologists Ford and Beach discovered in their remarkable study of a hundred and eighty-

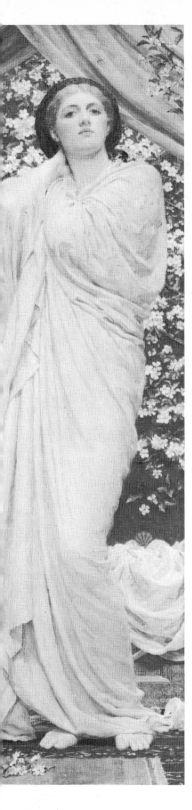

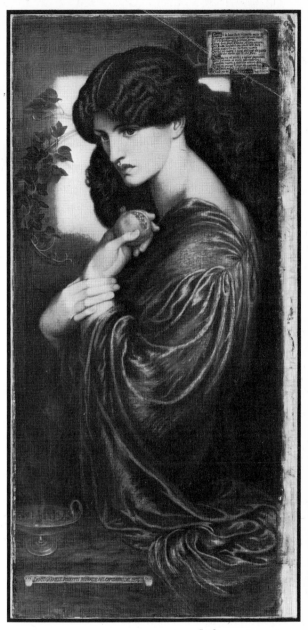

Left:
Blossoms *Albert Moore, 1881*

Right:
Prosperpine *D. G. Rossetti, 1874*

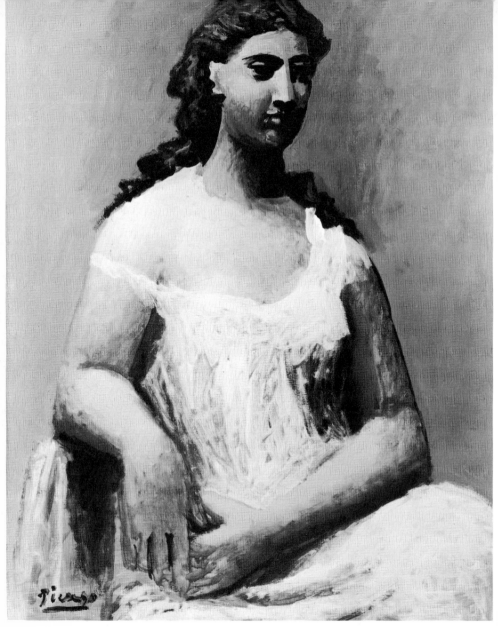

Seated woman
Picasso, 1923

five different societies that it was invariably the familiar, well-known, and, most important of all, the *well-understood* girls who were judged the most beautiful by the men. Exotic, unusual girls might have been fascinating to watch from a safe distance, but it always seemed to be the girls whose ways were understood who were chosen in the end.

But our standards of beauty arise from familiarity of another kind—the familiarity we have with the person in the mirror. As Ambrose Bierce once put this point:

Admiration: our polite recognition of another man's resemblance to ourselves.

There is no question that narcissism is deeply ingrained in our natures; we like people with our own characteristics, mental or physical. Boardrooms, in consequence, tend to be populated by images of the Chairman. And, of course, the process works both ways: those who are like us like us.

It is quite clear that beauty involves very much more than the possession of particular bodily features. Beauty certainly cannot be equated with sexual attractiveness. Nor can it be described simply in mathematical or geometrical terms. The truth of the matter is, as the Scottish philosopher David Hume realised more than two hundred years ago, that beauty is essentially a private and personal experience. 'Beauty,' he said, 'is not a quality in things themselves; it exists merely in the mind which contemplates them; and each mind perceives a different beauty.' He utterly rejected the old Greek view of beauty as something which could be defined in terms of physical shape and proportion. Beauty depends absolutely and completely on the eye and mind of the beholder. The weight of all the evidence collected over the last two hundred years seems quite firmly on Hume's side. Eric Newton surveys much of this evidence in his book *The Meaning of Beauty,* and finds himself in complete agreement with Hume. Beauty is something which causes man pleasure. But what causes pleasure to one need not necessarily cause pleasure to another; the criteria of pleasure and beauty are entirely personal. If there is any agreement about the beauty of a particular person it merely reflects the common experience of those who agree; such agreement does not imply, however, that any objective standard of beauty exists. And, as we have seen in an earlier chapter, anthropologists have shown beyond all doubt that ideas of beauty vary from society to society; standards are extremely variable and highly local.

The Italian philosopher Croce brought us perhaps even closer to the truth when he demonstrated that it is *in our minds* that the people we see before us are created. 'Every portrait artist,' he said, 'paints not the person before him so much as the person in his mind.' When we are offered a face to view we do not measure its proportions, or assess its

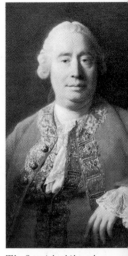

The Scottish philosopher David Hume (1711–76) believed that beauty was a highly individual experience created entirely in the mind of the beholder. Portrait by Allan Ramsay

details objectively. We do not compare it with some universal, or even local, ideal We use it as a convenient framework on which to hang our personal feelings, our momentary impulses. The face we create 'out there' is merely a vehicle for our personal projections, which spring from a multitude of internal causes. A significant proportion of every facial impression is created from within ourselves. Now this has an important consequence, so far as the purely visual aspect of beauty is concerned. As students of perception have long been aware, the less distinct the thing we are looking at, the greater will be the contribution from within the perceiver's own mind. It follows therefore that the more *indistinct* the face we see, the more chance will it provide of supporting our personal projections of beauty. The Impressionist painters were aware of this old principle—their paintings gain much from their lack of clarity and distinctness. It is interesting to see how, in the modern cinema too, this same principle of ambiguity operates. Many popular film beauties seem to have a curious capacity to portray each man's conception of beauty—different as this no doubt will be for each man in the audience. The box-office returns confirm that these stars succeed in supporting the maximum number of personal fantasies. This leads us to the interesting speculation that the most popular and successful film beauties, acting ability aside, will be those with the most enigmatic faces: faces which can be all things to all men—saints, mistresses, professional supports—whatever indeed passion or ambition desires. Even more successful at the box office will be those rare film faces which show promise also of satisfying not only the varied, but also the *fluctuating,* needs of man's fantasy life—the mother, the saint, the witty hostess in the morning, the warm seductive temptress at night. Herein perhaps lies the peculiar appeal of stars of genius, like Bergman and Garbo. Their faces have an exquisitely 'convertible' quality that can sustain the wildest—and the most diverse—fantasies. No need for soft camera lenses here, no need for tricks of lighting. There is a seductive ambiguity inherent in their faces, and so much more besides. Their whole *being* seems vague, indefinite, and unstructured—infinitely flexible and malleable to man's every need. Theirs is the ultimate in 'facial convertibility'.

Opposite
Garbo: 'a face infinitely convertible'

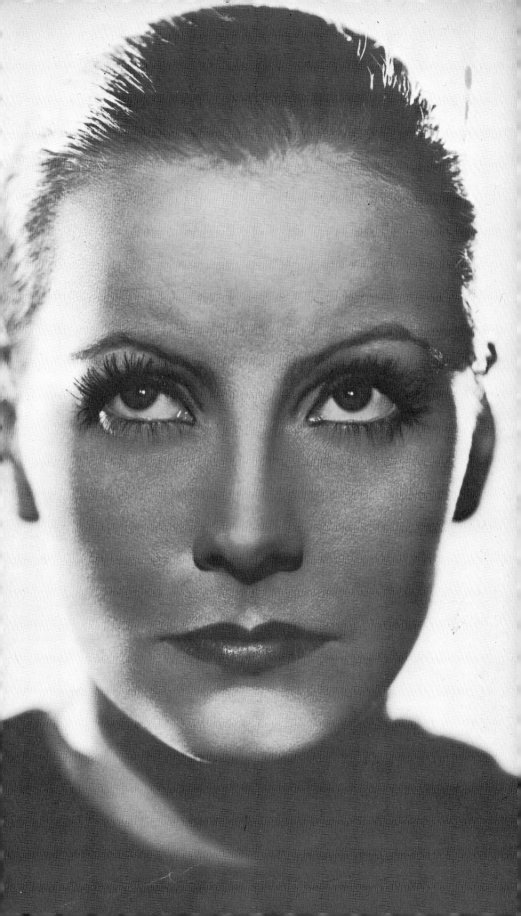

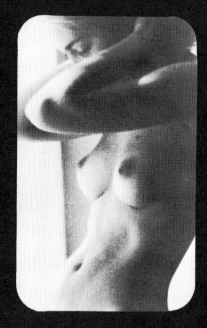

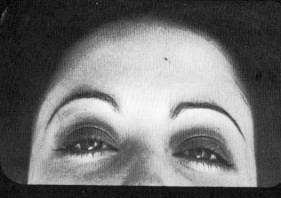

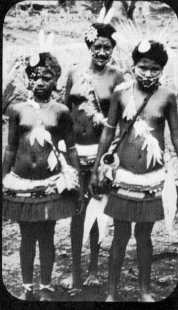

'If it were the fashion to go naked,' Lady Mary Wortley Montagu once declared, 'the face would be hardly observed.' But she was wrong. As anthropologists have consistently found, naked peoples find the greatest possible interest in the faces of their companions. Even more surprisingly, the face often seems to provide for them a major focus of erotic interest. Indeed, as Malinowski discovered, the naked Trobriand Islanders of the Western Pacific devoted much more energy to the decoration and elaboration of the face than to any other part of their bodies, except perhaps for the decorative tattooing of older girls around the vagina, which was simply the local sign for sexual maturity. It was the eyes, particularly, which were, for the Trobrianders, 'the gateways of erotic desire'. A source of great delight, known as 'Mitakuku' was the biting-off of eyelashes during lovemaking:

A lover will tenderly or passionately bend over his mistress's eyes and bite off the tip of her eyelashes. This, I was told, is done in orgasm as well as in the less passionate preliminary states.

But the nose, too, ranked almost as highly in erotic importance. It should be full and fleshy but not too large; it should be a 'standing-up' nose. It should not be aquiline, which was considered ugly. A flat nose was a serious blemish, whether in male or female, and severely limited sexual opportunities. The mouth and lips, too, were important; indeed they played a vital part in the Trobrianders' love-making, the shape of the lips in particular being regarded as crucial for sexual attractiveness. They should be full, but well-shaped and 'well cut'; protruding lips were considered almost as unattractive as pinched or thin ones. The 'ugliest possible was a drooping lower lip'. The lips are, of course, among the most highly sensitive regions of the body and it is easy to see how emotional excitement may arise from the lightest tactual stimulation. Desmond Morris believes they serve also as important *visual* signals in love-making—that their bright colour contrasting against neighbouring pale skin calls attention to the availability of an erogenous zone. He argues that sexual arousal produces a swelling and reddening of the lips—a change which itself constitutes an important sexual signal that serves to create

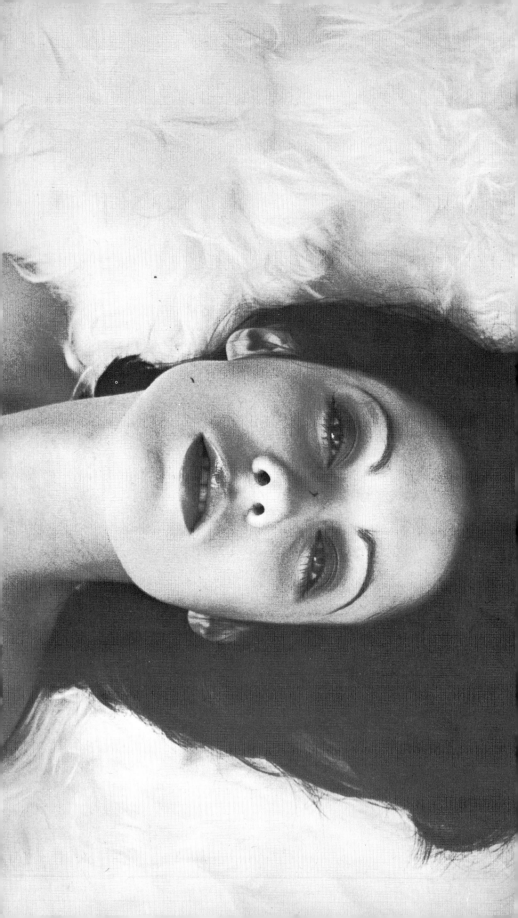

yet further excitement. In dark-skinned peoples, he says,
'what they have lost in colour contrast they have made up
for in size and shape.' This perhaps explains the characteristically large 'everted' shape of the lips among negroid
peoples. There are other parts of the face, however, which
are richly supplied with sensory nerves and which play an
important part in love-making. The lobes of the ears, for
example, have become sensitised to erotic stimulation;
indeed, according to Morris, this is their major purpose.
They are not, in his view, 'useless fatty excrescences', nor
are they remnants of primitive times when man had big ears,
as anatomists have sometimes claimed:

It seems that, far from being a remnant, they are something new, and when we discover that, under the influence of sexual arousal, they become engorged with
blood, swollen and hypersensitive, there can be little
doubt that their evolution has been exclusively concerned
with the production of yet another erogenous zone.

According to Morris parts of the nose perform a similar
function:

. . . the side walls of the nose contain a spongy erectile
tissue that leads to nasal enlargement and nostril expansion by vaso-congestion during sexual arousal.

And there are yet other parts of the face which play a
crucial part in love-making, as Morris explains:

By making tiny movements of the flesh around the mouth,
nose, eye, eyebrows, and on the forehead, and by re-
combining the movements in a wide variety of ways, we
can convey a whole range of complex mood-changes.
During sexual encounters, especially during the early
courtship phase, these expressions are of paramount
importance.

But it is not only in sexual encounters that the face assumes
such high importance. In ordinary everyday social life, of
course, it plays a central part. Its role is crucial in greeting
and in declarations of salutation and homage. There are
some curious examples of ceremonial greeting to be found.
In the Phillipine Islands the custom used to be to greet
newcomers by rubbing the guest's hand or foot over the
host's face. An old Nigerian form of greeting was to kneel
and rub foreheads together. Rubbing of noses, too, is a

Opposite *Desmond
Morris has described the
many visual signals
which arise from the face
during lovemaking*

Lips: *bright colour and
swelling calls attention
to erogenous zone*
Lobes of ears: *become
swollen and hyper-
sensitive*
Side walls of nose:
*contain erectile tissue
leading to nasal enlarge-
ment and nostril
expansion*
Mouth, nose, eye-
brows, forehead:
*small flesh movements,
combined in a variety of
ways, convey important
courtship signals. Pupils
dilate during sexual
arousal. Eye surface
glistens*

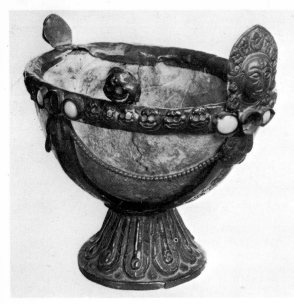

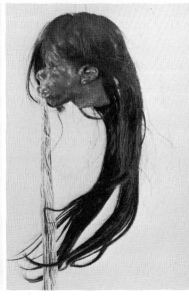

not-uncommon form of greeting. The original purpose of this is said to have been to allow two people to experience the scent of each other's body; this was accounted the most highly intimate mode of contact possible.

Among the Trobrianders, as Malinowski discovered, the face and head were held to be sacred, and for that reason often quite untouchable, especially in the case of persons of high social rank and importance:

> The sanctity of the chief's person is particularly localised in his face and head, which is surrounded by a halo of strict taboos. More especially sacred are the forehead and the occiput with the neck. Only equals in rank, the wives and a few particularly privileged persons, are allowed to touch these parts, for purposes of cleaning, shaving, ornamentation and delousing.

And the sacred significance of the face did not end with death of the body. In many lands and in many historical times, the face and head of the dead have often been regarded as especially sacred. Even today, a lock of hair may carry a peculiar significance as a remembrance of a loved one. But in some parts of the world it was the custom to keep far more than a lock of hair; in Tibet and Bhutan the whole head was severed from the corpse, and preserved as a treasured reminder of the dear departed. The body itself was usually put out to birds of prey but the head was always

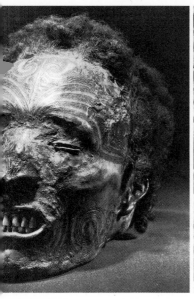
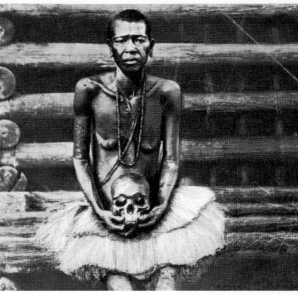

preserved as a sacred household treasure. Among the Indian peoples of Benares a similar practice once prevailed. Magical powers of protection were often attributed to such severed heads. Herodotus tells that in ancient times the slain heads of vanquished enemies were displayed before the conqueror's house because of 'their magical power to protect the whole house'. Goethe tells how he saw dried heads at the gates of his home city. And this old belief persisted until quite recent times in Stockholm where the heads of executed criminals were displayed outside the city.

It was the magical power of the head and face which so fascinated the head-hunters of Borneo, because, as they believed, the adversary's spirit was contained within his head. How better to conquer the spirit than by chopping off the head? The Indians of North and South America, too, treasured and preserved the faces and heads of their enemies. Even today this practice of head-hunting and head-shrinking continues among the Jivaro Indians of Equador, despite official prohibition. It is interesting to see how the mouths of these shrunken faces have been tightly sewn up 'to prevent the spirit from escaping'. Head-shrinking is undertaken by removing the bones of the skull and then alternately soaking, kneading and drying the skin, all the while taking care to preserve the facial features. A fine collection of such trophies from former times can be seen in the ethno-

Left *The intricately tattooed heads of famous chieftains were often mummified by the Maoris and held in great reverence and respect. Many examples survive from the 18th century*

Right *Trobriand widows of the late 19th century carried their husbands' skulls to the end of their lives*

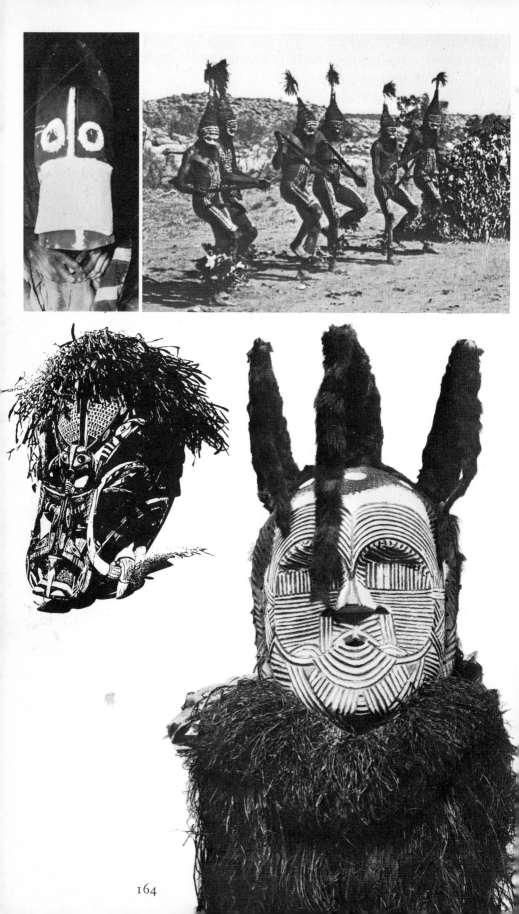

ogical museum at Guayaquil in Equador. Shrunken faces are proving a great success in the tourist industry of South America, though it is quietly understood that most of those generally offered for sale now are in fact made from monkeys, whose faces, when appropriately shrunken, present a strikingly human appearance.

The notion that spirits reside in the head has suggested to many peoples that the best way of curing a man who was mad or possessed of evil spirits or devils was by drilling or 'trephining' a hole in his skull to allow the evil spirit to emerge. Archaeologists have shown that such trephination has been practised for many thousands of years. And, given this belief that spirits reside behind the face, primitive man found it natural enough to construct representations of his gods and his spirits in facial images. These idols formed a useful focus for his spiritual activities. Thereafter it was but a small step from *making* a god to *becoming* one; by wearing the appropriate facial image, or better still, by *enclosing* oneself in it, all of its magical powers could be acquired. This explains the significance and popularity of masks among primitive peoples.

Masks have many advantages to be exploited. Their proportions and features can easily be exaggerated, and the effect can be exciting. Deliberate distortions can be introduced to disturb the onlooker. Fearsome details, such as the teeth or skin from a lion, can be added, which will not only frighten the enemy but confer on the wearer, by magic, the lion's power and ferocity. Masks are not the static objects of wood and straw we see in ethnological museums: they are dynamic, moving objects which play a crucial part in complex ritual occasions composed of dance, chant and ceremony. The most impressive masks are, without question, those whose features are hard to discern—where it is hard to decide, perhaps, whether there are two eyes—or four—or eight, whether the mouth is open or closed—or whether, indeed, there is any mouth at all. Skilfully constructed, such masks may acquire a tantalising ambiguity. Their continual fluctuation from one apparent facial form to another leaves the observer spellbound; they hold the attention much more powerfully than could any realistic facial representation. And their effect is all the more impressive when they are

Opposite:
Top left *Mask of Akuma: a cult object also worn and danced in. Julcon Benue Province, N. Nigeria, 1930*

Top right *A daylight ceremony. The ambiguity —and so the influence— of masks is much increased if they are seen at night by flickering firelight when conditions for perception are poor*

Bottom left *An infinity of fluctuating faces, figures and mysterious creatures can be created by the mind from this highly ambiguous Sepik mask. Malanggan cult object from New Ireland*

Bottom right *This Congolese mask, like many other ritual masks, combines elements which are life-like and realistic with elements which are fantastic, mysterious and quite unreal* seen in flickering firelight. It is in just these conditions, of course, that masks are most frequently used, because it is at night that the spirits are believed to be especially active.

Masks have many distinct uses; they can preserve life and cure ills, especially in the hands of the tribal medicine man or *feticheur*. The more frightening and mystifying he makes his mask, the more effective will be his treatment, especially in those disorders which are largely psychological, and which western medicine chooses to describe as 'hysterical'. In old African communities the *feticheur* combined the function of physician, magistrate and priest. The distinctive mask which he wore served to enhance and confirm his importance; it concealed his miserably ordinary personal identity and created for him an entirely new and powerful personality. Like a uniform, it defined his role and confirmed his status. He became, by common consent, the embodiment of all the spirits enshrined in the folk-beliefs of the tribe and was converted, at least temporarily, into a potent spirit commanding instant obedience and respect. In Ceylon, the medicine men used different masks for each separate disease and affliction. The illustrations show a mask used to cure deafness, another for bronchial complaints, and another to cure stammering. In Java, on the other hand, they used their medicine masks rather differently: here they served as protective charms against disease, rather than as cures.

The curious power of the facial image over the imagination is clearly shown by the central part which masks and idols have always played in religious celebration and in the ceremonials of death. In ancient Egypt masks were believed to be capable of conferring eternal youthfulness on the deceased; they ensured for ever his welfare in the next world. The splendour of some of these funeral masks can be seen in the golden mask of Tutankhamun. In ancient Greece, masks representing Persephone, goddess of the underworld, were often attached to the faces of the dead to protect them, and to ease their journey into the next world. In tombs at Mycenae such funeral masks have been discovered, beautifully fashioned from gold. Masks of great beauty were worn too, in religious ceremonies, by the worshippers of Apollo and Dionysus. But in time these ceremonies deteriorated into festivals of great revelry, the

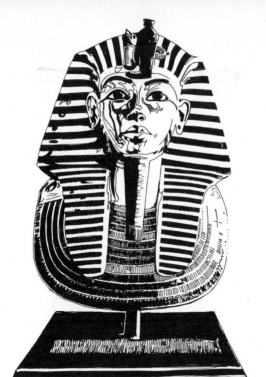

*The most famous of all
death masks: the
funerary mask of
Tutankhamun, made
from solid gold, glass
and precious stones*

*A beautifully-preserved
solid gold funerary
mask from Mycaenae*

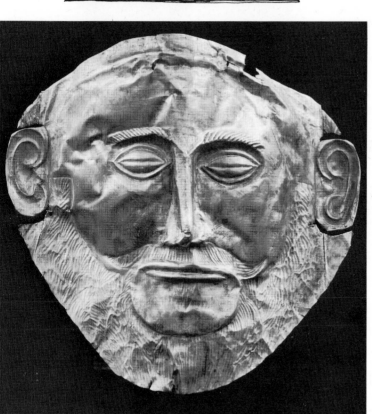

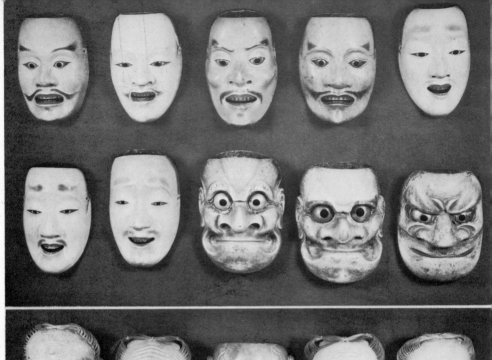

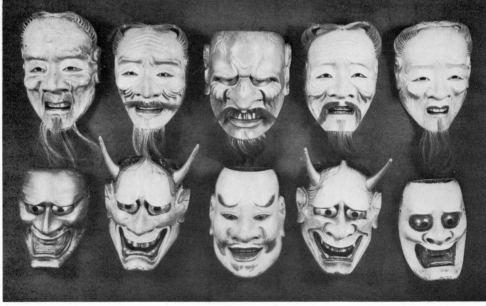

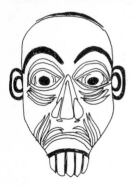

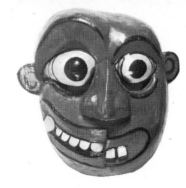

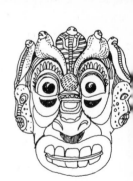

wearers of the masks taking full advantage of their anonymity to engage in riotous orgies. Grotesque and amusing variants of the old religious masks also became popular, and the revellers began to play 'parts' appropriate to their masks. In this way the mask gave birth to dramatic art. Different colours were used to denote heroes and villains; masks became increasingly sophisticated and eventually quite large, so that the action could be followed in the great amphitheatres even though the players' words might not be audible.

Masks virtually disappeared from the civilised world after Roman times, but reappeared in the Middle Ages in the Mystery plays which became popular throughout Europe as a form of religious entertainment. Colourful masks are employed even today in Eastern Asian Mystery plays. And Japan, China, Tibet, Burma, Thailand, Ceylon and Java each have their own characteristic theatre in which masks play a crucial part. In the 'Bunraku' and 'No' forms of theatre, which still flourish in Japan, curious and pleasing effects are achieved by surrounding the impassive masks by elegant movement and gesture. Recent research has discovered an interesting and hitherto unsuspected property of the face-mask: somehow, it seems, the mask may alter the personality of the wearer, at least temporarily. Of course, it has long been realised that a shy, middle-aged partygoer can be transformed into a youthful Casanova by giving him a simple false nose. But it has only recently been discovered that the wearer of a mask makes facial-movements *behind* the mask appropriate to the character represented. Possibly this accounts for the effectiveness of the theatrical mask; perhaps it encourages in the actor feelings, postures, gestures and expressive movements appropriate to the character he is portraying.

It is evident that masks are highly *versatile* objects. They can be beautiful objects in their own right. They can perform duties in religion, magic, healing and war. They can entertain and they can amuse. They can generate, particularly when used in social gatherings, emotion and excitement of considerable intensity and, as anthropologists believe, they can even help unite whole societies. Finally, as we have just noted, they do seem to be able to change the

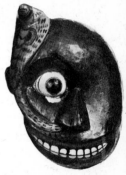

A painted wooden mask worn by devil dancers of Ceylon to cure deafness

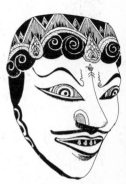

A wooden mask used in Javanese 'Topeng' drama in the 19th century

Opposite:
Top 'No' Theatre *masks from Japan*

Left *A Ceylon devil-dancer's mask used for the cure of bronchial catarrh*

Centre *A strangely asymmetrical mask from Ceylon used for the cure of stammering*

Right *Devil dancer's mask from Ceylon*

experience of those who wear them. But why are they so strangely effective? Part of the explanation lies in their unreality. We are always fascinated—sometimes even disturbed —by faces which are changed, distorted or disfigured. There is a curious ambivalence towards such departures from the familiar: we must look again and again. We find ourselves fascinated by even slight deviations from the 'correct' pattern. Somehow, it seems, the pattern of the face has become so deeply etched in our mind that any departure, however slight, is unsettling.

There is no more convincing proof of the hold of the face over man's mind and imagination than the volume, variety and ubiquity of folk-legends involving the face. The same themes occur again and again in stories which have fascinated generation after generation the world over. The eyes feature particularly frequently: tales have been told for thousands of years of single-eyed gods like Odin, and powerful Cyclopean monsters with one amazing eye in the centre of their forehead. Tales have long been told, too, of strange men with mysterious powers who had three, four or, in the case of one story, even six eyes. In Chinese legend there were men with 'doubly-powerful' eyes with two pupils, and in Irish tales there were eyes which had three and even seven pupils. There have been tales of eyes which flicker with burning coals or flash with lightning. Countless stories have been told about eyes containing all-consuming serpents which devour all they look upon. Devils, too, were said to inhabit the eyes, particularly those of witches— although less important hags have often had to make do with cats or dogs. Tales of the 'evil-eye' occur in all cultures. Among the Ibo of Nigeria there are tales about noses and mouths and eyes which actually *move about the body*. There are even legends about whole faces which can be moved about the body and even 'lent out' to other people, and there are stories, now linked with customs among some tribes, of 'face-throwing', in which the spirit residing in the face can be 'thrown' across the intervening space to influence the other person for good or ill.

Mystics have sometimes suggested that parts of the face have symbolic significance. For the ancient Egyptians, the eye symbolised 'the power and the perfection of

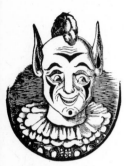

One of the infinite faces of Harlequin. Wood-cut from Victorian Delights

Opposite *Old Japanese theatrical mask*

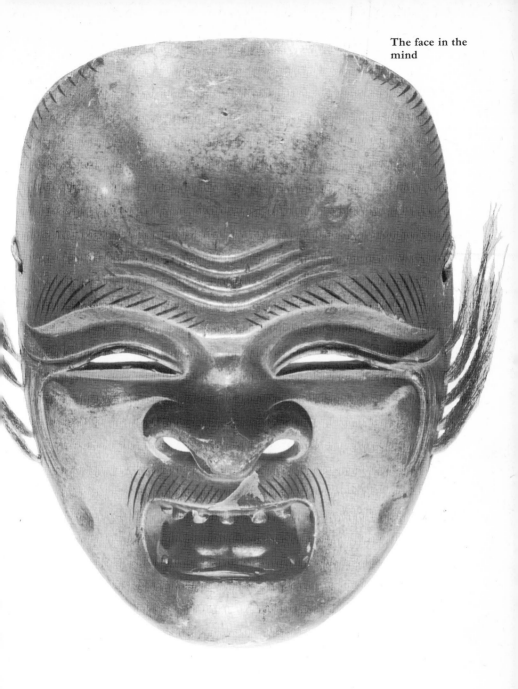

the sun'. The perfect circles of the pupil and the iris contained between the lids represented, according to one writer 'power under control'. Another interpretation was that they represented 'the sun in the mouth'. To Jung, the eye symbolised 'the rest and peace of the maternal bosom'. But speaking in this way of the features of the face as 'symbols' does not help us to understand the underlying processes of thought, since anything can be taken to symbolise anything; the important question is why were these facial features chosen? Extra eyes were once believed to confer extra spiritual power: to have two eyes was normal, to have three was superhuman or divine. And eyes which appeared in unusual parts of the body—'heterotopic' eyes—were believed to confer spiritual insight and power on that particular bodily part. There are many legends of such eyes bringing strange new powers to hands, legs, torsos and arms, as well as various unusual parts of the head. Such heterotopic eyes were once common in paintings of fantastic beings, angels and deities.

The mouth is well represented in folk-legend, especially those breathing fire. The 'all-consuming fiery mouth' is often mentioned in ancient literature; it is frequently represented as the royal road to the terrible underworld. Psychoanalytic writers have often dwelt upon the unconscious significance of the mouth, sometimes suggesting that it is associated in the mind, albeit unconsciously, with the female genitalia. In support of this idea they cite not only the free-associations of their patients but also strange legends like those of the vagina-dentata, the toothed mouth-like vulva, which bites off the husband's penis. Some psychoanalysts are convinced of our continuing pre-occupation with the mouth for quite another reason, namely that it is a constant reminder of our very first important contact with the world outside ourselves—our mother's breast. The nature of much of our subsequent personality development depends, they say, on our happy or unhappy experiences during these early contacts. There are many jokes about the mouth, just as there are about the face generally, and jokes, like dreams and recurring legends, are known to be useful guides to the contents of the deeper layers of the mind. One legend tells the tragi-comic story of the wry-mouthed family in which each member fails in turn to blow out the candle before bed. In another version, each of them fails to drink the magic potion that would make their mouths normal again.

The hair figures prominently in folk tales. The awesome event of forcible cutting-off of hair has been celebrated with great gusto in the tales of many lands. Lamps have been lit with the moustaches of monarchs, and fur hats made from the beards of conquered Welsh Kings. Here was the final insult, the highest indignity. The Bible, of course, tells how Samson's 'strength went from him' after Delilah had 'shaved off his seven locks of his head.' Psychoanalysts believe these tales are so persistent and so exciting just because the hair is associated, albeit unconsciously, with sexual activity. And cutting it off, they suggest, may very well symbolise something much worse: castration.

Tales of unusual noses, bent or hooked or long, like Cyrano de Bergerac's, have always been a source of fascination. Large noses have often been represented in such tales as indicating virility, an idea which, as we shall see, occurs again and again in the writings of the old physiognomists. Modern psychoanalytic writers are not in the least surprised by this notion—it is something else which recurs, they say, with almost monotonous regularity in the free associations of their patients undergoing analysis. Some therapists even declare that the nose is somehow associated, in the deep layers of the mind, with the penis.

One of the most interesting and remarkable characteristics of the human mind is its unceasing capacity to generate images and ideas. Sometimes these images seem to be created out of the air; nothing tangible is needed to bring them into existence. But this creative act is not restricted to the realm of thought: it extends beyond thought to visions. We can create visions of things which in reality have no existence. And even when we are looking at real objects our ever-creative minds are capable of modifying them in quite remarkable ways. There is often only the most tenuous link between 'what we see' and 'what is there'. The disparity is even more marked in conditions where things can be only dimly seen—where outlines are vague and indistinct. Dimly-lit church interiors, misty

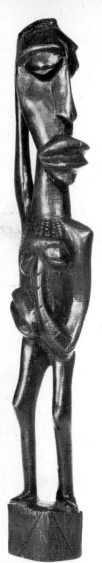

moorlands, dark forests—these are the places where the mind plays tricks, where the mind transforms reality, making us see things which are not physically present. The correspondence between appearance and reality is likely to be all the less if we are under strain, or fatigued or fearful, or when we are driven by some strong need or desire. All too often we see what we want to see rather than what is truly there. It is curious how often, under conditions such as these, we see a face. The image of the face seems to take precedence over all others when the visual scene is at all unclear. The face seems to be, for all of us, a 'preferred shape'. We can see faces in the fire, faces in rocks, faces in clouds—faces in the moon. Scrooge even managed to see Marley's face in his own door knocker. It is strange to discover, too, how artists, designers of hardware—even builders of grottoes as our illustration shows—seem to be impelled, in their creative work by this same hidden image of the face. Many seemingly 'abstract' decorations often contain strong facial shapes, though often enough their designers were probably genuinely unaware of this influence.

Just why the face should constitute such a powerful basic 'schema' for our experience is an unsolved mystery. Is it perhaps the earliest shape we had to learn outside ourselves? Does every baby have to learn the all important shapes of his mother's face as his first lesson in survival? Or is there something perhaps even more basic in the geometry of the face? Does its overall shape—or the disposition of its separate parts—remind us, however dimly, of something else: the whole body perhaps? It is true that there is a curious parallel—as artists like Magritte have not hesitated to show us—between the patterns of the face and the patterns of the whole torso. Magritte makes breasts into eyes and the pubic region into a mouth. African artists, in their masks and statues, constantly provide echoes and re-echoes of this same strange confusion. With curious skill they fascinate our attention with breast eyes and vulva-mouths and, sometimes also in male figures, with penis noses and tongues. The power of these sculptures is often enhanced by the delicacy and skill with which this ambiguity has been introduced by the artist and by the way in which the details have been given continuously oscillating

Much primitive art provides evidence of the confusion in the deeper layers of the mind between the imagery of the face and the imagery of the torso: a Kenyan wood-carving

Opposite *Facial imagery in architecture: the Villa Orsini in the Parco dei Mostri at Bomarzo uses eyes and nostrils for light and a mouth as the great entrance doorway*

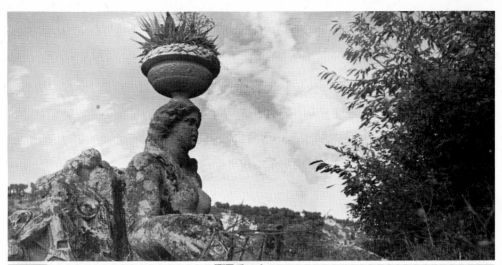

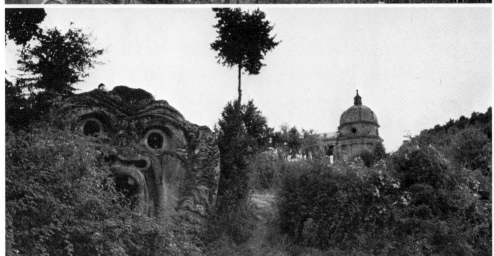

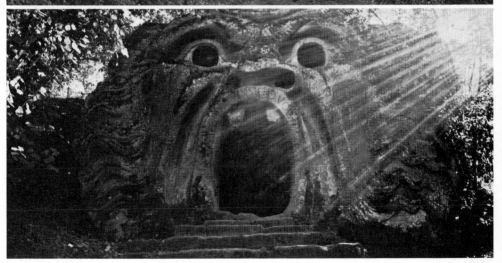

175

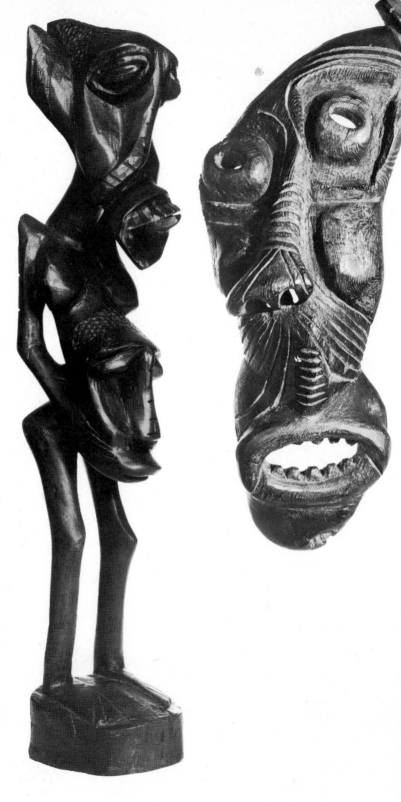

Left *Another Kenyan wood-carving providing further evidence of confusion between the imagery of the face and that of the torso*

Right *The distortions and ambiguities of this carving encourage a rich variety of bodily imagery in the mind of the perceiver*

Opposite *The artist often provides new insights into the workings of the mind.* The Rape *by Magritte*

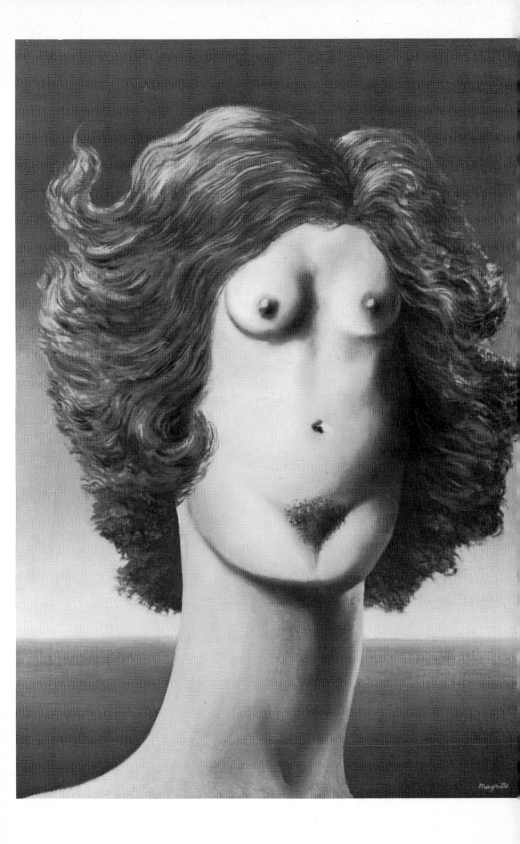

meaning. These mental confusions come as no surprise to psychoanalysts who have long been convinced of the sexual significance of nose, eyes, mouth and tongue. But the paintings of Magritte, the African sculptures, and even ancient sculptures such as the 'Venus of Willendorf' suggest there is a more primitive and profound association in the mind between the whole, integrated pattern of the face, and the pattern of the torso. There is indeed a curious congruence between the geometry of the face and the geometry of the torso. Perhaps this is why the facial pattern has come to be such a 'preferred form' and why it takes such precedence in conditions of difficult perception; perhaps the face represents something which is biologically of supreme importance in perpetuating the species, the human body itself.

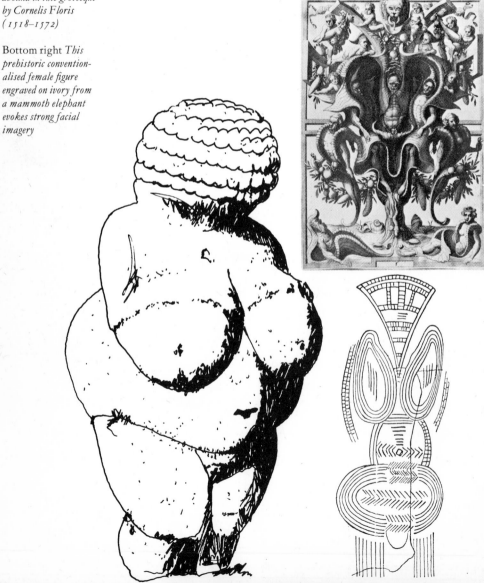

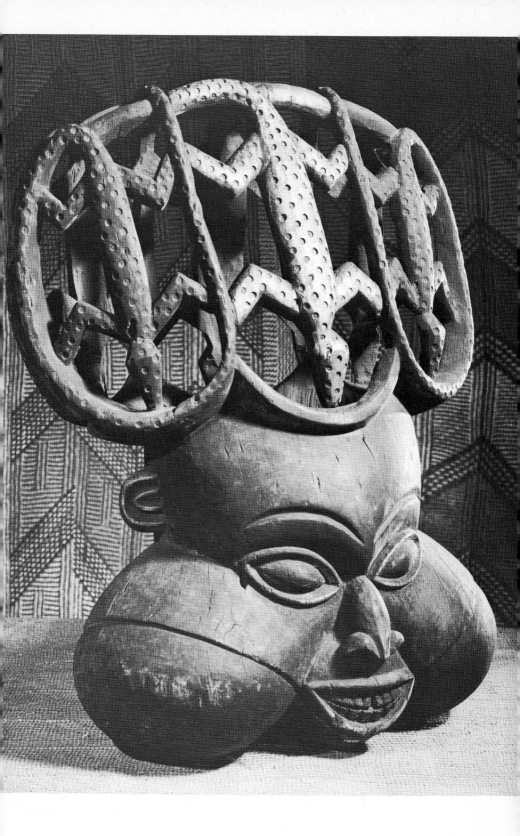

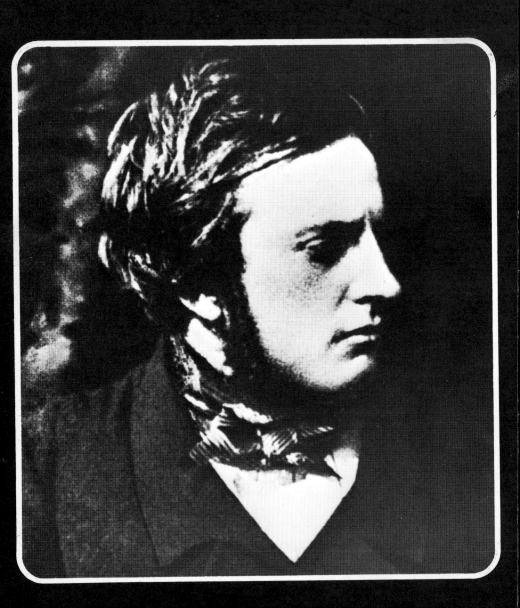

The belief that character can be 'read' from the face is as ancient as it is widespread. It is reflected in old proverbs about the dangers of people with squints and sparkling eyes. It can be found in the Bible and in the works of ancient philosophers and poets. The seventeenth century Jesuit scholar Niquetius named no less than a hundred and twenty-nine of the great scholars of classical Greece and Rome who had written at length on this subject—among the philosophers and theologians were Aristotle, Plato, Seneca and Tertullian; among the historians, Xenophon, Plutarch, and Tacitus; among the poets, Aristophanes, Juvenal, Lucian and Petronius; and among the naturalists and physicians, Hippocrates, Celsus, Galen and Pliny the elder. Pythagoras is known to have regarded physiognomy very seriously indeed; he allowed no student into his academy to study mathematics unless his facial appearance showed that he could profit from his teaching. According to Plato, Socrates did likewise and admitted no scholar to philosophy unless he was quite sure by examining the student's face that he was suited to it. Aristotle devoted six chapters of his *Historia Animalium* to the study of facial appearance, and described the signs of such qualities as strength and weakness, genius and stupidity, timidity and impudence. He declared, for example, that

> Men with small foreheads are fickle, whereas if they are rounded or bulging out the owners are quick-tempered. Straight eyebrows indicate softness of disposition, those that curve out toward the temples, humour and dissimulation. The staring eye indicates impudence, the winking indecision. Large and outstanding ears indicate a tendency to irrelevant talk or chattering.

A large face, according to Aristotle, was the sign of meanness, whereas a small face was 'steadfast'. A broad face was 'stupid', whereas a round face was the sure sign of courage.

But to Hippocrates, the 'father of medicine', the face was primarily the indicator of health or disease; it was of the greatest utility as a practical diagnostic aid. He described for the first time the most fateful face of all—the drawn and pinched *facies Hippocratica*—the face of those about to die. Polemon, a physiognomist of the second century, did much to bring respectability and popularity to physiognomy by

Guides to character ?

Opposite *How different physiognomists might have read this photograph by Octavius Hill*

Concave nose= *Forbearance, imagination* Lavater

Forehead perpendicular= *Great intellect* Aristotle

Eyebrows close to eyes= *Earnest, deep firm character* Lavater

Long brows= *Faculty for the sciences* Hill

Indent in middle of chin= *Cool understanding* Lavater

his character descriptions of contemporary leaders, which were eagerly sought. In fact, 'face reading' became firmly established as an honoured profession in classical times. In the great days of Imperial Rome, the Romans needed no convincing of the relationship between face and character; for them the faces of the marble portrait busts arranged around their courtyards seemed the very embodiment of the greatness of their ancestors. But there were other faces they collected, much stranger than these. There developed in Roman times the curious cult of the 'Imagines'—the collecting of wax death masks, which they proudly displayed in their homes and carried in family funeral processions to proclaim to all the world the excellence of the character of the departed. As Pliny explained in his *Natural History*, there were two activities which had been regarded as indispensable for every good Roman citizen in former and more glorious times: the maintenance of a family archive and the keeping of a family tree. He chided his contemporaries for their lack of concern for art, and for their neglect of treasured portraits of ancestors:

> In the halls of our ancestors it was otherwise; portraits were the objects displayed to be looked at . . . and wax models of faces were set out, each on a separate sideboard to furnish likenesses, to be carried in procession at family funerals.

He described how the death-masks or 'Imagines' were taken from the corpse and incorporated into terracotta busts. Unattractive though they were, they served an important purpose as a constant reminder of the strength of character of the departed. This curious death-mask cult had a strange but short-lived revival in Florence in the fifteenth century—and many curious and unappetising specimens from this time are still to be seen.

A thousand years after Roman times the Arabian philosophers Averroes and Avicenna were still extending and developing the ancient teachings of Aristotle. Avicenna explained the art of character judgement in *De Animalibus*. The Persian physicians Ali ben Ragel and Rhazev explained and developed Aristotle's ideas. But another three centuries were to pass before interest in this subject was to be awakened in Western Europe by Albertus Magnus, the

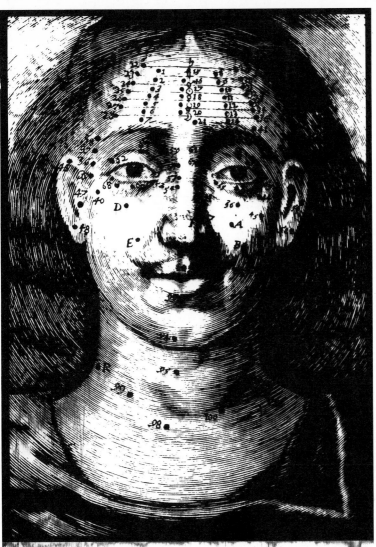

As recently as the 17th and 18th centuries, it was widely believed that the stars influenced the face as well as the character. This illustration from Cardarno's Fisionomia Astrologica *relates the signs of the zodiac to lines of the forehead*

teacher of Thomas Aquinas, who wrote on physiognomy in his *De Animalibus*. The first printed book on physiognomy was the work of Michael Scot, astrologer to Frederick II, *De Hominis Physiognomia*, which was written in 1272 and printed in 1477. This book attempted, probably for the first time, to provide physiological explanations of facial forms and expressions, and to discuss the action of specific nerves and muscles. Since it was written by an astrologer, however, its explanations were of an occult and magical kind. Indeed, physiognomy was to become, for the next five hundred years, hopelessly confused with the white magic of 'judicial astrology', by which fortunes could be

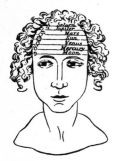

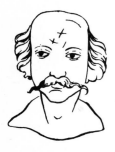

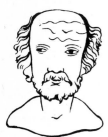

Top *Smooth forehead*
Middle *Drowning*
Bottom *Melancholy*

foretold and influences from the stars explained and pre-dicted. Books of this period, of which there were many, on physiognomy (or podoscopy or metaposcopy, as it was variously known) were filled with the strangest assertions. A single example from the work *Fisionomia Astrologica*, written by Cardano in 1659, will suffice. As the illustration shows, seven lines were drawn on the forehead held temporarily smooth. The upper line was the line of Saturn, then came Jupiter, Mars, the Sun, Venus, Mercury and the Moon. When the skin of the forehead was released to its natural form by removing the privileged and magical hand of the physiognomist the lines might remain straight or parallel or they might cross or lie obliquely. The possessor's character and future would be indicated by the way the lines settled. The lines of the second diagram predict that the man was doomed to die by hanging or by drowning. The third diagram shows the lines of a man suffering from melancholy. Whilst a great many books on physiognomy were published throughout Europe in the sixteenth cen-tury, Thomas Hill's *The Contemplation of Mankind*, written in 1588, was the earliest work on the subject printed in English. He described his book as 'a pleasant introduction to the art of chiromancie and physiognomie', and explained in it the art of discerning the four types of face, which were to be found associated with the four basic temperaments. As the Greeks had long ago explained, there were four basic 'temperaments'—the 'melancholic', the 'sanguine', the 'choleric' and the 'phlegmatic'—corresponding to the four basic 'elements' which made up the whole universe: earth, air, fire and water. In a popular work of the seven-teenth century *The Passions of the Minde in generall* Thomas Wright offered this advice on the facial colours to be looked for in the four 'humours':

To a red man, reade thy need:
With a brown man breake thy bread:
At a pale man draw thy knife:
From a black man keep thy wife.
The redde is wise,
The brown trustie,
The pale peevish,
The black lustie.

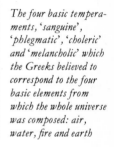

1. Sanguine *2. Phlegmatick*

3. Cholerick *4. Melancholy*

*The four basic tempera-
ments, 'sanguine',
'phlegmatic', 'choleric'
and 'melancholic' which
the Greeks believed to
correspond to the four
basic elements from
which the whole universe
was composed: air,
water, fire and earth*

Elizabethan dramatists like Shakespeare and Jonson employed physiognomical detail and interpretation so often
and so naturally that we cannot doubt that beliefs of this
kind were part of the common fund of knowledge in the
sixteenth and seventeenth centuries. Milton employed
physiognomic notions in *Comus* and in *Paradise Lost*: the
devil's facial appearance altered, for example, as his moral
nature was revealed. Dryden, too, tried to give his fictitious
characters convincing reality by describing them in currently
popular physiognomic terms. He also drew heavily upon
new ideas on the expression of the passions which Des-
cartes, Hobbes and Spinoza had recently expounded. A new
scientific spirit was in the air; new discoveries in anatomy
and physiology—like Harvey's discovery of the circulation

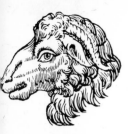

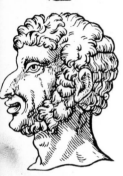

Della Porta was impressed by the similarity of man and animals. Goat-faced men, he believed, were like the goat, stupid

of the blood—were beginning to turn people towards a search for natural rather than magical and celestial causes. The attack on old-fashioned magical physiognomy began in 1627 in an important and highly popular work by G. B. Della Porta, *Of Celestial Physiognomy*. Throughout the six volumes of this book he attacked the falsehood of the old judicial astrology. Della Porta left his readers in no doubt that both character and facial features result from a man's temperament and not from the stars. After citing the opinions of astrologers on the character of men born under the influence of Saturn he declared:

> We have reported their opinions, not to approve of them but to refute them as old woman's stories. Dissimulating their falsehood, presenting as coming from heaven and the stars . . . they make us accept as divine that which is derived from natural sources.

He explained how, according to the astrologers, the Saturnians had been said to be 'melancholy cold and sapless' because of Saturn's power. But this was quite wrong; the words of Hippocrates the physician made it quite clear that melancholy, cold and saplessness are products of temperament—not of any celestial influence. The problem of character judgement, therefore, was that of discovering the varieties of temperament and the relationships between each of these and the features of the face. But then Della Porta went on to make some much less credible assertions which unfortunately have been linked with his name ever since. Important insights about temperament were, he said, to be obtained by making facial comparisons between man and animals. 'Goat-faced men, like the goat, were stupid.' 'Lion-faced men were, like lions, strong and fearless.' Della Porta, who is often thought of today as the great representative of all that is most foolish in ancient physiognomy, was, in fact, the initiator of a revolution of thought which was steadily, over the following two hundred years, to rid the study of physiognomy of its magical nonsense. Though there is little of permanent substantive value in his writings they had one highly important effect: they facilitated and encouraged the gradual introduction of a new, positive, scientific approach to the study of the face.

In 1697 the diarist John Evelyn wrote a *Digression*

concerning Physiognomy in which he gathered together seventeenth-century ideas on human biology and physiognomy. The 'spirits of the passions' he believed, resided in the medulla of the brain. By constant repetition of favourite passions or vices these spirits flowed ever more easily into particular nerves of the face, so that eventually the face became 'unalterably fixt'—displaying thereby the character of their possessor. Like Della Porta, he believed in the ancient doctrine of the four humours, and expressed the interesting view that a well proportioned face denoted a proper balance and proportion of the humours. He undertook an analysis in the *Digression* of famous contemporaries such as Bacon, Cromwell, Hobbes and Jonson. But, like Della Porta and so many others before him, he was bemused by the curious facial similarities of man and beast, and clung to terms such as 'sheepish', 'hog-jawed' and 'rabbit-mouthed' in his personality descriptions. He explained the significance for character of individual features. Of the forehead he said if it has 'too much swelling, and fleshy it betokens stupidity . . . if lean, subtlety; if narrow, indocile; if too round, unsteady; if convex and asinine, folly; if depressed, effeminate; if square and ample, lion-like in courage.'

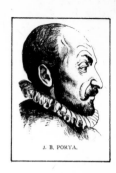

J. B. PORTA.

Popular interest in physiognomy persisted unabated throughout the seventeenth century and on into the eighteenth. Addison and Steele's *Spectator* of 1711 contained two papers on physiognomy, the first of which concluded that 'we may be better known by our looks than by our words . . . a man's speech is more easily disguised than his countenance.' The second was more of a satire, suggesting that physiognomy was at most a pseudo-science best left to enthusiastic amateurs. These papers reflect the intense popular interest of the subject in the early eighteenth century. The intelligentsia, too, were much concerned with physiognomy: Kant, for example, wrote a paper on *National Physiognomies.* Boswell reported his conversation with Rousseau (15 Dec. 1765) in which he himself declared, 'I am a physiognomist, believe me. I have studied that art very attentively, I assure you, and I can rely on my conclusions.' To this Rousseau replied, 'Yet I think the features of the face vary between one nation and another

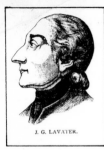

Johann Kaspar Lavater 1741–1801. Pastor, teacher, poet, and most famous of all physiognomists. Killed by a sniper's bullet while tending the wounded during the attack on his home town of Zürich

Opposite and following pages 191, 193, 194, 195, 197, 198, 202, 203 Lavater illustrated with his own fine drawings many men and women and explained in Essays in Physiognomy *how their characters could be deduced from their facial features. Modern psychologists do not accept his explanations*

as do accent and tone of voice, and these signify different feelings among different peoples.'

It was at this time, however, towards the end of the eighteenth century, that a remarkable man appeared, who was to dominate the whole realm of physiognomy for a century or more. He was Johann Kaspar Lavater, a pastor and teacher, the son of a physician in Zürich. He was a wise man, much loved and respected by his fellow citizens who, it is said, flocked about him in the streets to hear his words. He was a shrewd, sensitive man who cared much for the welfare of his fellow men; he had found his true vocation as spiritual guardian of his flock. But his gifts were many. He was a talented artist, and an indefatigable recorder of his acquaintances. It was from these drawings, and from his ceaseless and acute observation of his parishioners and neighbours that the system of physiognomy arose. He was certainly a gifted and astute observer of the face. He is said to have immediately recognised and correctly named the death-mask of Mirabeau the revolutionary—and this in an age when portraits were rare and photography, of course, unknown. In fairness, it must also be recorded that he mistakenly identified the portrait of an executed assassin as that of Herder, the German philosopher and poet, crying out, so it is said, in ecstatic delight over 'its intellectual and poetical qualities'. But perhaps the assassin was also a poet?

Lavater's great fame arose from his *Essays in Physiognomy*, which appeared in their earliest form in 1772 and quickly became immensely popular and translated into many languages. In the words of *The Gentleman's Magazine* of 1801,

> In Switzerland, in Germany, in France, even in Britain, all the world became passionate admirers of the Physiognomic Science of Lavater. His books published in the German language were multiplied by many editions. In the enthusiasm with which they were studied and admired, they were bought as necessary reading in every family as even the Bible itself. A servant would, at one time, scarcely be hired till the descriptions and engravings of Lavater had been consulted in careful comparison with the lines and features of the young man's or woman's countenance.

1 *A boldly sketched portrait of Albert Dürer*
Whoever examines this countenance cannot but perceive in it the traits of fortitude, deep penetration, determined perseverance, and inventive genius. At least everyone will acknowledge the truth of these observations, when made.

2 *Moncrif*
There are few men, capable of observation, who will class this visage with the stupid. In the aspect, the eye, the nose, especially, and the mouth, are proofs, not to be mistaken, of the accomplished gentleman, and the man of taste.

3, 4 *Johnson*
The most unpractised eye will easily discover, in these two sketches of Johnson, the acute, the comprehensive, the capacious mind, not easily deceived, and rather inclined to suspicion than credulity.

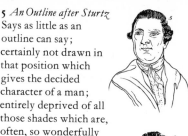

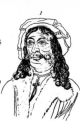

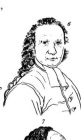

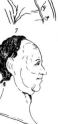

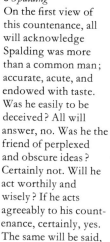

5 *An Outline after Sturtz*
Says as little as an outline can say; certainly not drawn in that position which gives the decided character of a man; entirely deprived of all those shades which are, often, so wonderfully significant: yet, if so rude an outline ever can convey meaning, it does in the present instance; and certainly, according to the physiognomical sensation of all experienced people, it is at least a capacious head, easy of conception, and possessed of feelings quickly incited by the beautiful.

6 *Spalding*
On the first view of this countenance, all will acknowledge Spalding was more than a common man; accurate, acute, and endowed with taste. Was he easily to be deceived? All will answer, no. Was he the friend of perplexed and obscure ideas? Certainly not. Will he act worthily and wisely? If he acts agreeably to his countenance, certainly, yes. The same will be said, whether viewed in front, or in profile, 7.
7 . . . the forehead, the eye, and the aspect, will appear, to the most uninformed, to betoken an elegant and reflective mind.

8 *Shakespeare*
A copy of a copy: add, if you please, a spiritless vapid outline. How deficient must all outlines be! Among ten

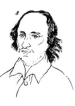

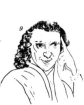

thousand can one be found that is exact? Where is the outline that can portray genius? Yet who does not read, in this outline, imperfect as it is, from pure physiognomical sensation, the clear, the capacious, the rapid mind; all conceiving, all embracing, that, with equal swiftness and facility, imagines, creates, produces.

9 *Sterne*
The most unpractised reader will not deny to this countenance all the keen, the searching, penetration of wit, the most original fancy, full of fire, and the powers of invention. Who is so dull as not to view, in this countenance, somewhat of the spirit of poor Yorick?

Even the sober *Encyclopaedia Britannica,* in its eighth edition, found itself impressed with Lavater's *Physiognomy*:

> Its publication created everywhere a profound sensation. Admiration, contempt, resentment and fear were cherished towards the author. The discoverer of the new science was everywhere flattered or pilloried; and in many places, where the study of human character from the face was an epidemic, the people went masked through the streets.

The early editions of the *Physiognomy* in Germany, France and England, were beautifully produced, with fine engravings. The purchaser of Lavater's book acquired, if nothing more, 'a picture gallery executed by some of the leading painters and engravers of the century and containing admirable likenesses of many of the famous figures of the day.' Subsequent editions, of which there have been a great many, have failed to match these early editions—whose printing Lavater supervised himself—in the quality and brilliance of their production and illustration. After nine successful German publications in the 1770s and 1780s there was a French translation which brought the work to an even wider audience and led to two English editions— one of which was the beautiful Henry Hunter translation costing thirty guineas a set. By the 1780s at least twelve English versions had appeared. By 1810 sixteen German, fifteen French, two American, one Dutch and at least twenty English versions had been printed. And the work was regularly reprinted until the 1870's, a hundred years after its first appearance. Two modern editions were produced in Switzerland in the 1940s which brought the total to 151 publications in all languages.

Lavater became much sought after by the great and famous and in the years following the publication of the *Physiognomy*. He was regularly visited at his home in Zürich by travellers from afar. The Emperor Joseph II consulted him in 1777, and later the Grand Duke of Russia, as well as Prince Edward of England.

But why was his work so popular? Perhaps because it promised a set of rules which could be learnt quickly— applied quickly? Or perhaps because he seemed to reach the correct conclusions so often? Who could doubt a

10 *S. Clarke*
Perspicuity, benevolence, dignity, serenity, dispassionate meditation, the powers of conception and perseverance, are the most apparent characteristics of this countenance. He who can hate such a face must laboriously counteract all those physiognomical sensations with which he was born.

11 . . . As is the full face, so is the profile; how emphatically does this confirm our judgement! To whom are not this forehead and this nose the pledges of a sound and penetrating understanding; this mouth, this chin, of benevolence a noble mind, fidelity, and friendship.

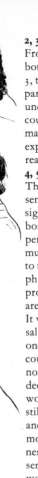

2, 3 *Two Fools, in profile*
From the small eyes in both, the wrinkles in 3, their open mouths, particularly from the under part of the countenance of 2, no man whatever will expect penetration, reasoning, or wisdom.

4, 5 *Two Fools*
That physiognomical sensation, which, like sight and hearing, is born with all, will not permit us to expect much from 4, although, to the inexperienced in physiognomy, the proper marks of folly are not very apparent. It would excite universal surprise, should any one, possessing such a countenance, pronounce accurate decisions, or produce a work of genius. 5, is still less to be mistaken, and I would ask the most obstinate opponent of physiognomical sensation, whether he would personally declare, or give it under his hand, that the man who expects wisdom from this countenance is himself wise.

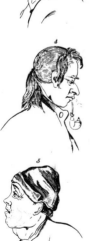

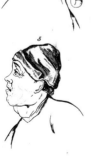

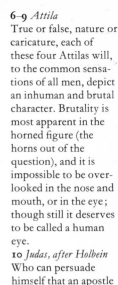

6–9 *Attila*
True or false, nature or caricature, each of these four Attilas will, to the common sensations of all men, depict an inhuman and brutal character. Brutality is most apparent in the horned figure (the horns out of the question), and it is impossible to be overlooked in the nose and mouth, or in the eye; though still it deserves to be called a human eye.

10 *Judas, after Holbein*
Who can persuade himself that an apostle of Jesus Christ ever had an aspect like this, or that the Saviour could have called such a countenance to the apostleship? And whose feelings will be offended when we pronounce a visage like this base and wicked? Who could place confidence in such a man?

system enabling him so rightly to conclude—from 'pure physiognomical sensations'—received from Shakespeare's portrait—that the poet had 'a clear, capacious, rapid mind; all conceiving, all embracing, that with equal swiftness and facility imagines, creates, produces . . .' And Lavater's work contained many more impressive analyses, together with beautiful drawings, of many other great figures of the past.

His objective was clear, and the title he chose was characteristic: to promote the love of man for his neighbour through the realisation of the beauty of the mind and the spirit—a beauty so clearly made by God and so clearly visible in the face, if only one took the trouble to look. There was no hint of judicial astrology here, no fortune-telling, no reliance even on simple theories of 'humours': simply an attempt at naturalistic description—an attempt to do for physiognomy what Linnaeus had done for botany—to produce a system of classification which would lead eventually to the formulation of hypotheses, and perhaps even laws, concerning the relationships between face and mind. His concern was to show the relationship of natural cause and effect—and to deny the mystical causes and occultism of earlier books on the subject, which he so deplored. Lavater, though clearly unimpressed by the works of earlier physiognomists such as Aristotle and Della Porta, quite modestly saw himself as nothing more than a blundering beginner in a new and daunting scientific enterprise. He constantly warned his readers of the difficulties and pitfalls of the new science—and utterly rejected those incompetents, ignorant of general principles, who carelessly and improperly undertook 'This most difficult of all studies . . . to the utter degradation of physiognomy.'

He considered the body to be composed of three divisions corresponding to the three major aspects of life:

The animal life, the lowest and most earthly, would discover itself from the rim of the belly to the organs of generation, which would become its central or focal point. The middle or *moral life* would be seated in the breast, and the heart would be its central point. The *intellectual life*, which of the three is supreme, would reside in the head, and have the eye for its centre. If we take the countenance as the representative and epitome

1–4 All will perceive in the four countenances of 1 to 4, fear mingled with abhorrence.

5–8 As with 1 to 4, in the four following, 5 to 8, as visibly will be perceived different graduations of terror, to the extreme.

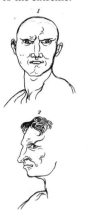

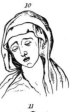

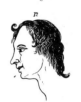

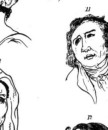

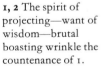

9–16 A succession of calm, silent, restless, deep, and patient grief, are seen in 9 to 16.

9–12 No man will expect cheerfulness, tranquillity, content, strength of mind, and magnanimity, from 9 to 12.

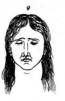

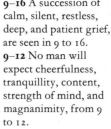

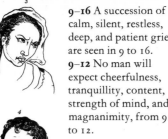

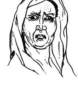

13, 14 Fear and terror are evident in 13, 14.

15, 16 Terror, heightened by native indocility of character.

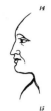

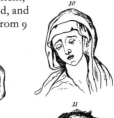

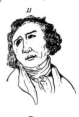

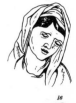

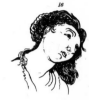

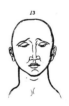

1, 2 The spirit of projecting—want of wisdom—brutal boasting wrinkle the countenance of 1.

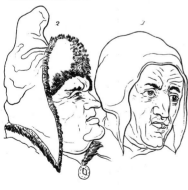

2, is the image of blood-thirsty cruelty; unfeeling, without a trait of humanity.

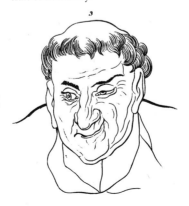

3 Virtue, noble simplicity, goodness, open confidence, are not discoverable here. Unbounded avarice, unfeeling wickedness, knavery unequalled, in the eye and mouth, eradicate every pleasing impression. It is possible this countenance might not have looked much better previous to its degradation, but vice only could produce the full effect we behold.

1 Calm wisdom, circumspection, simulation, a phlegmatic-melancholic temperament. All is unity almost extraordinary, almost superior, yet neither; clear, unconfused, not inventive; quick of perception, not creative; active in thought, but not courageously progressive.

2 A caricature of one of the noblest, firmest, most thoughtful, and sensible countrymen. The stability of the original is in this outline become obstinacy; the penetration of the eye censorious acuteness; and the fortitude of the mouth contemptuous severity; still is it a compact, original character, and worthy to be studied; easily persuaded to uncommonly daring actions, but not to evil.

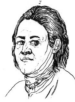

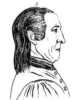

3 Who could believe that this is the same countenance; in the former, too sharply, here too timidly, drawn? Both penetrating, acute, rapid, not to be deceived. The forehead in this has most understanding and capacity for instruction; the mouth most honest industry; the nose most benevolence. The whole speaks one language and I dare affirm that the original is one of the most sincere, thoughtful and friendly men that is to be found among the peasantry of Switzerland.

4 Another farmer of unwearied industry; wise to begin, courageous to pursue, and patient to complete. This head is formed much to comprehend and much to undertake; this eye to reflect. The nose is full of practical prudence. The mouth less eloquent than persuasive; the chin, the wrinkles are characteristic of rapid activity.

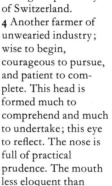

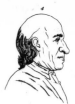

5 A farmer of Zürich, from the opposite part of the country; rather rough than strong, voluble than eloquent, imitative than inventive, insinuating than powerful; labouring more from necessity than choice; apter to collect than to distribute, to desire than to enjoy.

6 A countenance which has the same relation to the former as the ideal has to the caricature. All is here more regular, noble, decided, reflective, unalterable. How much more pure is the forehead; more simple, more thoughtful, the eye how much softer! The nose is more patient, not so choleric, but, separately considered, appears to have less mind than the former. This mouth, this chin, are incomparably more desirous to return affection than the former.

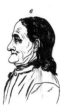

7 Another countryman (mentioned in the first part of Meiner's Letters on Switzerland) and one of the most thoughtful and acute we possess; of a phlegmatic-melancholy temperament; not only accurate in proof, but deep in research; full of calm, admiring sensibility for all that nature contains of truth and greatness. Considered separately, the nose appears to have no character, but, united to this forehead, maintains its worth. Beneath this powerful eyebrow rests a steady, unconstrained, penetrating eye. The whole countenance has the expression of calm, faithful, firm, wise, inoffensive activity.

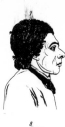

8 A faithful, discreet, innocent, wise, clear, mild, modest, well-judging countenance, of an indefatigably industrious Zürich farmer, in which the traits all appear to harmonize in favour of faithful benevolence and propriety.

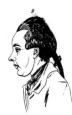

9 The profile of a young countryman of Zürich, full of youthful simplicity, innocence, good nature, and good sense; who is now a man, and has formed himself after, and preserved the national character, in all possible perfection. This head, one of his first performances, appears to bear a like proportion to his present works, as the countenance here given does to his present countenance; the same free accuracy brought to perfection: the same clearness, assiduity, and disgust for everything that is merely manner; for everything obscure; the same greatness of taste, and infantine simplicity.

10 A very expert tradesman: the countenance unspeakably decisive, to the very point of the double chin, for activity and discretion. It is really astonishing to see how many prudent, expert, experienced, I am almost tempted to say, incomparable, country people we have. The cavity that will be formed, if a line be drawn from the end of the nose to the chin, and that occasioned by the descent of the forehead to the nose, are traits that, decisively, speak practical prudence.

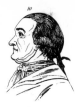

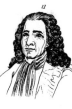

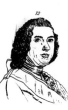

11 The delicate construction of the forehead, the aspect of the man of the world, the beauty of the nose, in particular, the somewhat rash, satirical mouth, the pleasure-loving chin, all show the Frenchman of a superior class. The excellent companion, the fanciful wit, the supple courtier, are everywhere apparent.

12 Another very different and more firm and thoughtful Frenchman. The upper part of the countenance to the end of the nose seems almost English; the under has the national sanguine of the French. The eyebrows in an Englishman would certainly be more firm, compressed and shaded; in other respects I love and esteem such countenances much.

of the three divisions, then will the forehead, to the eyebrows, be the mirror or image of the understandings; the nose and cheeks the image of the moral and sensitive life; and the mouth and chin the image of the animal life; while the eye will be to the whole as its summary and centre. It cannot however too often be repeated that these three lives, by their intimate connection with each other, are all, and each, expressed in every part of the body.

All men are impressed by the faces they see, Lavater insisted, and cannot help drawing conclusions from what they see in them. The scientific physiognomist, on the other hand, could learn his craft only by careful, diligent observation and laborious comparison. But the effort was worth while, for the fruits of such training were considerable, and of inestimable value to prince and judge alike, to parent, guardian and teacher, so that they might properly evaluate the abilities of children, and so assist their proper fulfilment. Lavater distinguished *physiognomy,* which he took to be the study of the implications of the static features of the face— the face in repose—from *pathognomy,* the study of the effects of 'character in motion', 'the knowledge of the signs of the passions', which he believed could, by repetition, leave their permanent mark. But the true physiognomist's task was clear—to study the relatively unchangeable elements of the face: the shape of the nose or the forehead or the colour of the eyes. Lavater was himself keenly interested both in physiognomy and pathognomy:

> The original dispositions are most discoverable in the form of the solid and prominent parts; and their development and application in the flexible features.

The correspondence of face and inner state was part of God's work, according to Lavater. God provided both the internal state and the correct external form to reveal that state clearly and honestly to mankind. There was no deception in the cosmic scheme; appearance *was* reality. His great concern was to discover the nature of these external signs which he sincerely believed were most clearly visible in the face. He wrote chapter after chapter on the implications of the fine detail of the face:

> The nose is the indicator of taste, sensibility and feeling;

Outline of eyes after Le Brun

1 Insipid, vacant, unnatural. The upper line may either belong to the eyelid or eyebrow.

2 Terror and wrath, devoid of power. The arching of the eyebrow and the breadth of this bony nose are alike impossible where the corner or angle of the eye is so obtuse.

3 Terror, abhorrence, and rage; but general, not determined, not accurate.

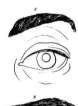

4 Eyes which never can attain the power of thought. The first outline of ignorant astonishment. Eyes which nothing take and nothing give.

5 Convulsive rage; the affectation of power without the reality.

6 Stupid devotion mixed with pain.

7 The eye of the choleric temperament, full of courage and active resolution.

8 Less courageous, but wiser; less firm, but more considerate. The angle of the eye is too short for an eye so long; the under bending of the upper eyelid not suitable to, not in congruity with the eyebrow.

9 With more genius than the former; but the angle again too obtuse, and the outline of the under eyelid inaccurate. An eye that penetrates the heart; entirely observant of men, and born heroic.

10 Less genius. The under outline, once more, inaccurate, unmeaning. A sanguine-phlegmatic eye; somewhat languid; rather considering the whole than attending to the minute; despising the little and disposed to the comprehensive.

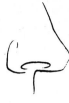

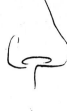

1–4 We may if we please reduce noses to three principal classes:

1 Those the under parts of which, or the nostril, including the lowest outline, may be considered as horizontal. These are the most beauteous, noble, and full of spirit. But they are very uncommon.

2 Those the under outlines of which, including the nostril, are turned up. These are commonly more low and hollow near the root than the example here given, in which the nostril is inaccurate, and the outline very noble.

3 The hooked nose, which usually denotes melancholy, and is, at least, seldom seen without a mixture or inclination to melancholy: or without wit, satire, and mind; to which, as a 4th we may add the cartilaginous, irregular, intelligent, determined, powerful, choleric nose.

9, 10, 11 Three very wise, acute, active noses, which we discover so to be by the undulations and gentle inflexions of the outlines.

9 is the most judicious, great and enterprising;

10 more mild, less choleric.

11 the least noble, though not ignoble; the most difficult to be deceived; the most acute.

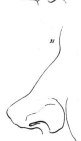

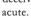

1, 2 Two imperfectly drawn outlines of mouths of very opposite characters; 1, seems to me the mouth of the refined, intelligent, eloquent man of taste, and of the world; the politician; 2, the dry, firm, close, immoveable, authoritative, phlegmatic, melancholy character.

3, 4, 5 Three—wherefore may we not say muzzles? (N.B. the distinction between the words mund and maul [or muzzle and mouth] have a propriety in the German which is lost in translation—T.)

Muzzles only appertain to beasts, or brutal men —how much are we the slaves of the works of our own hands, and of the breath of our own mouths! How continually do we forget that speech was made for man and not man for speech. I will therefore venture to say three mouths, 3 and 5, belong to one class, and are nearly of the same character: mildly discreet, peaceful, humble, attentive.

4 has more power, is more concentrated: has more esteem, less affection; is more pertinacious, more resolute.

6–9 Not one of these four mouths is natural; 7 is the most so, and is alone benevolent, acute, capacious, tender, affectionate, noble, peaceable and loving order.

6 is altogether as brutal as a mouth can be, in which we suppose any acuteness and satire. The upper part of 7, has something crafty the under, rude and stupid. The upper lid of 8 participates of goodness, but the under is as weak, as toneless as possible.

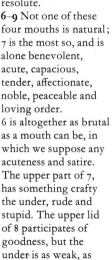

the lips mildness and anger, love and hatred; the chin the degree and species of sensuality, the neck the flexibility, contraction, or frank sincerity of the character; the crown of the head, not so much the power as the richness of the understanding; and the back of the head the mobility, irritability and elasticity.

Like so many other physiognomists before and since, he accorded pride of place to the forehead, which he continually praised and subjected to minute analysis. On the significance of the forehead many physiognomists seem to have been able to agree. Even the great nineteenth-century anatomist Sir Charles Bell found himself in complete agreement with Lavater:

> The forehead is more than any other part characteristic of the human countenance. It is the seat of thought, a tablet where every emotion is distinctly impressed; and the eyebrow is the moveable type for this fair page.

Lavater's chapters are full of signs to be diligently sought. Consider, for example, the signs in the eyes:

> Eyes which are large, open and clearly transparent, and which sparkle with rapid motion under sharply-delineated eyelids—always denote five qualities: quick discernment, elegance and taste, irritability, pride, most violent love of women.

Again, the 'signs' to be found in the nose:

> A woman with a deeply concave root of the nose, a full bosom, and a somewhat projecting canine tooth, will, notwithstanding her homeliness and unloveliness, more certainly, more easily, and more irresistibly lead away the whole herd of grovelling voluptuaries than a perfect beauty. The worst prostitutes brought before the spiritual courts are always of this conformation. Avoid it as a pestilence, and form no connection with any such—not even a matrimonial union, though the reputation be apparently unblemished.

It was this sort of uncompromising and unqualified advice which so powerfully attracted the attention of his readers. Even wrinkles told us the truth:

> Oblique wrinkles in the forehead, especially when they are nearly parallel, or appear so, are certainly a sign of a poor, oblique, suspicious mind. Parallel, regular, hori-

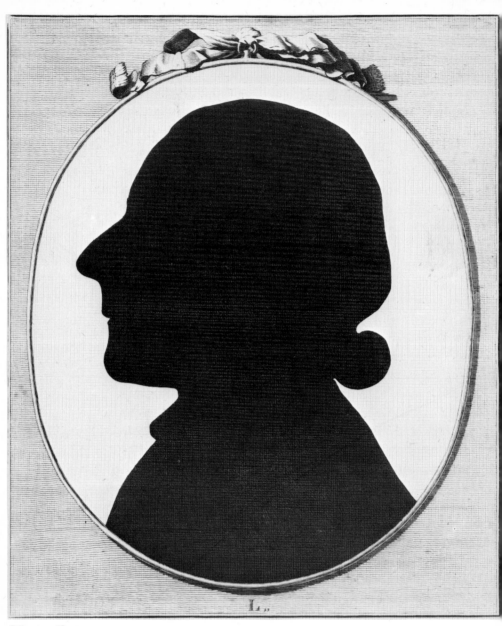

Silhouette of Lavater

zontal, not too deep wrinkles of the forehead, or parallel-interrupted, are seldom found except in very intelligent, wise, rational and justly-thinking persons.

Lavater had much to say on children's faces. He declared some quaint beliefs about the appearance of children, and some of these persist even today—for example, that the mother's imagination affects the physical appearance of her child: '. . . from the imagination of the mother, comes sensibility, the kind of nerves, the form and the appearance.' 'We know that children most resemble the father only when the mother has a very lively imagination and love for or fear of the husband.'

He had some interesting ideas too, on the similarity of lovers:

If a man deeply in love, and supposing himself alone, were ruminating on his beloved mistress . . . it is probable that traits of the mistress be seen in the countenance of this meditating lover.

It has, of course, frequently been suggested that those who spend a great deal of time together grow alike—that we all become like our friends, that teachers become like the children they teach—and even that dog-lovers, to some degree, become like their dogs. Again, according to Lavater, a man ruminating on his hatred for another might very well, for a time, take upon himself the hated man's appearance:

So might in the cruel features of revenge the features of the enemy be read. And thus is the countenance a picture of the characteristic features of all persons exceedingly loved or hated.

One of the most serious and persistent errors of Lavater, like so many other physiognomists, ancient and modern, is the error of 'metaphorical generalisation'—the argument from 'straightness' of feature to 'straightness' of character, from 'obliqueness' of brow to 'obliqueness' of character. Even 'roughness' of hair, eyebrows and skin he declared to indicate 'roughness' of character. This kind of association, a favourite device of physiognomists, dramatists and novelists alike, is, alas, without the slightest shred of justification.

And there is a further disabling flaw which runs throughout his work; he was almost completely ignorant of the

1 Corrupt rudeness, and malignity, condemning morals. Natural power degenerates into obstinacy, in the forehead. Affection is far distant from this countenance. Insensibility usurps the place of courage, and meanness the seat of heroism. Alas! what must thy sufferings be ere thou shalt be purified equal to thy original destination! The thing most pitiable in this countenance is an expression of the conscious want of power to acquire the degree of malignity it may wish, or affect to possess.

2 How much too vulgar, too mean, is this form of countenance for the great, unique, the incomparable Luther, who with all his monstrous faults, if so you shall please to affirm, still was the honour of his age, of Germany and of the human race! This form of countenance, I say, is nothing less than beautiful; yet may every half observer discover the great, the firm, the fearless man—What mind, what enthusiasm in the eye and eyebones! What industry and humility in the mouth! For in such situations, with such incitements to pride, who was more humble? It were needless to notice the inflexibility and power of the chin, and the neck.

3 The most accurate female housewifery: the forehead entirely feminine; the nose indicative of household discretion; the eye sharply attentive; the mouth kind, but strictly economical; the undulation of the jawbone as effeminate as possible; all the wrinkles express good sense, confined within a small domestic circle.

4 Noble, full of vivacity, youthful frolic, sanguine, capable of friendship, innocent, mild, faithful, modest, and in the outline of the nose, especially, charming effeminacy.

5 More power, comprehension, sensibility, desire of instruction, capacity, practical reason, combined with the most faithful friendship and punctual love of order. Forehead, eyebrows, eye, nose, and mouth—all one mind, one character.

6 The forehead less, the other features all more feminine than the former. The forehead and nose have something masculine, which gives a beautiful support to the mild, cheerful, noble sanguinism of the other parts.

7 How much heroism is there in this caricature! The form of the forehead, though feminine, is as manly as a female forehead can be. How conspicuous in eyebrow, eye, nose, mouth and chin, are faith, worth, and the incorruptibility of the noble character!

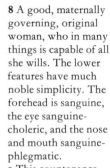

8 A good, maternally governing, original woman, who in many things is capable of all she wills. The lower features have much noble simplicity. The forehead is sanguine, the eye sanguine-choleric, and the nose and mouth sanguine-phlegmatic.

9 This countenance contains more than might be suspected. The forehead has clear and capacious understanding: astonishingly acute, virgin perception in the nose; mild eloquent diction in the mouth and chin; distinguishing love in the religious eye. The remaining features natively cold and dry.

10 Forehead, eye, nose, and mouth, individually, are expressive of a capacious and extraordinary woman. If this forehead does not easily receive and restore with additions, if this nose does not produce something uncommon, and if this eye has not its moments of genius, then will I renounce all pretensions to physiognomy.

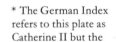

*11 Except the smallness of the nostril and the distance of the eyebrow from the outline of the forehead, no one can mistake the princely, the superior, the masculine firmness of this, nevertheless feminine, but fortunate, innocent, and kind countenance.

* The German Index refers to this plate as Catherine II but the

sovereign of all the Russias was so well known that the Editor probably thought it would be superfluous to write her name under her portrait.

Socrates

According to this head, after Reubens, which we shall first consider, Socrates had certainly great propensities to become eminent. If he resembled this copy, and I have no doubt but that his appearance was better, for this may be the twentieth copy, each of which is less accurate, the declaration of Zopyrus, that he was stupid, was incontrovertibly erroneous; nor was Socrates less mistaken when he was so ready to allow that he was by nature, weak. It may have been, and perhaps was, an inevitable effect of the weight of these features, that the perspicuity of his understanding was, sometimes, as if enveloped by a cloud. But had Zopyrus, or any true physiognomist, been accustomed accurately to remark the permanent parts of the human face, he never could have said Socrates was naturally stupid.

Whoever considers this forehead as the abode of stupidity, has never been accustomed to observe the forehead. If Zopyrus, or any other ancient, has held this arching, this prominence, or these cavities, as tokens of stupidity, I can only answer they have never been accustomed to consider or compare foreheads. How great soever the effects of a good or bad education, of fortunate or disastrous circumstances, and whatever other influence, of better or worse, may become, a forehead like this will ever remain the same, with respect to its great outlines of character, and never can escape the accurate physiognomist. In these high and roomy arches, undoubtedly, the spirit dwells which will penetrate clouds of difficulties, and vanquish hosts of impediments.

The sharpness also of the eyebones, the eyebrows, the knitting of the muscles between the brows, the breadth of the nose, the depth of the eyes, the projection of the pupil under the eyelid, how does each separately, and all combined, testify the great natural propensities of the understanding, or rather the powers of the understanding called forth! And how inferior must this twentieth or thirtieth copy be, compared to the original! What painter, however good, is accurate in his foreheads? Nay, where is the shade that defines them justly? How much less an engraving from the last of a succession of copies!

'This countenance, however, has nothing of that noble simplicity, that cool, tranquil, artless, unassuming candour, so much admired in the original. Something of deceit and sensuality are clearly perceptible in the eye'.

In the countenance before us, yes; but a countenance of this pregnancy and power may exert an astonishing degree of force in the command of its passions, and by such exertion may become what others are from a kind of imbecility; and further, I affirm the living countenance may have traits too evident to be mistaken, which yet no art of the painter, no stroke of the engraver, can express. This subject was lightly mentioned in a former fragment: I here repeat, with a greater degree of precision—

The most disgusting vices are often concealed under the fairest faces; some minute trait, inexpressible by the graver, to be seen only occasionally, when the features are in motion, will denote the most enormous vice. Similar deceptions are found in a distorted, or rather in a strong and pregnant countenance; such as is that of Socrates. The most beauteous, noble, and active characteristics of wisdom and virtue, may discover themselves only by certain indefinable traits, visible to a spectator when the features are in action.

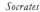

Socrates

anatomy and natural history of the face. His work contains many simple errors of physiological fact. The keenness of his eye was not enough to make up for his ignorance of natural history. His writing contains wholly unsubstantiated assertions about the functional significance of the features of the face.

Attacks on his system were made from many sides—by rationalists who disliked his mysticism, as well as by those of methodical mind who were frustrated in their search for a coherent system or set of principles by which to judge character. Certainly, the reader will look in vain for general guiding principles, because the works of Lavater contain none. Perhaps this was due to his genuine concern not to oversimplify what he recognised to be a difficult subject. When, at the end of the eighteenth century, interest in the physiognomy was at its height, a number of satirical letters were published in *The Gentleman's Magazine*. It was not so much the detail of Lavater's writings they attacked as the whole proposition that character could be read from the face. In particular, his comparisons of men and animals came in for much ridicule.

There was a brisk and famous controversy between Lavater and his contemporary Lichtenburg, who wrote a vicious but entertaining lampoon on the subject of 'reading character from dogs' tails'. But Lavater remained quite unmoved; there was no hint of bitterness in his 'reply'. There were many other detractors, however—among them the cartoonist Gilray. Isaac Disraeli also published a brilliant satire, *Flim-Flams*, in 1806, in which not only Lavater but Camper and Erasmus Darwin were castigated for their foolish 'scientific' excesses. Lavater was satirised, too, on the stage as 'Lord Visage', in an early nineteenth-century farce, *False Colours*, but was stoutly defended in a review of the play by Holcroft, his English translator. In another play of 1848, however, *Lavater: the Physiognomist or Not a Bad Judge* his image had evidently mellowed, for he was represented as a warm, benevolent man of towering ability. A French vaudeville of 1848 even cast Lavater as the scientist-hero who unmasked the villain by skilfully reading his face. William Sotheby, in 1790, went so far as to write a poem in which physiognomy was presented as an exact science.

Early in the nineteenth century an American, Joseph Bartlett, wrote a poem which seemed to raise Lavater almost to the status of a direct instrument of God. Referring to the serpent and the fall of man, he wrote:

Had but Lavater's science then been known,
We had been happy, Paradise our own:
Eve would have seen the craft, which lurk'd within,
Perceived the Devil . . .
Then this our earth Millenium had been,
Free from all death, from misery and sin . . .

Lavater was no more, but certainly no less, successful than those who were to follow him over the next two hundred years in trying to describe in clear, unequivocal terms the relationships between facial form and personality. He did not achieve a system of explicit, rational rules—although he constantly implied that such general principles did in fact exist. His analyses were intuitive. But his descriptions were all too often merely rhapsodies, pleasant to hear, but empty of meaning. His work is important nonetheless, not so much for the new insights it provided, for there are few, but because it brought to an end forever the old mysticism and magic in which almost all earlier works on the face had been deeply immersed.

His work had a pleasingly 'scientific' flavour much in tune with contemporary interest in science; Lavater made more than passing reference to newly acquired knowledge in the increasingly fashionable sciences of anatomy, zoology, physiology and anthropology. His work was doubly attractive, because he was a sincere man, a devout man of God, who seemed to be offering a reassuring resolution of the disturbing conflict becoming ever more apparent between scientific and religious ideas. And it is interesting to see that Lavater refused to consider or discuss evil.

At the beginning of the nineteenth century there arose a strange new pseudo-scientific movement which was soon to achieve enormous popularity. This was the study of 'phrenology', which was concerned with the precise shapes and contours of the head and the relationship between qualities of character and prominences on the skull. The Viennese physician F. G. Gall believed that the brain consisted of a number of separate and distinct 'organs' or 'centra' which could develop independently and to a different degree in different people. As these special areas grew and developed they produced their own swellings or bumps on the skull which could be seen and felt from the outside of the head. Since each of the 'centra' corresponded to a 'faculty' or to a quality of temperament it therefore became possible, Gall maintained, by feeling a man's skull, to decide which of his faculties were well-developed, and which under-developed. There were, he believed, twenty-seven of these separate cerebral 'organs', each corresponding to a particular 'faculty'. A well-developed protuberance of the forehead, for example, would indicate well-developed 'mirthfulness'—whereas a prominence on the back of the head would indicate 'amativeness'. Another important faculty, the intellectual faculty of 'causality', was located in the upper forehead. As Gall eagerly demonstrated, the faces of Socrates, Bacon and Galileo all showed this to a high degree. Another intellectual faculty, the faculty of 'comparison', made its own characteristic bump, which again he showed to be particularly prominent in the heads of Kant, Chaucer, Locke and Michelangelo. And if further proof were needed of the validity of Gall's theory, he went on to show that the head of Rossini (which he had personally examined) had an especially well-developed bump corresponding to the faculty of 'tune'. The busts of Haydn, Gluck and Mozart also showed each of them to be well-endowed in this respect. Gall urged, however, that caution be observed in arguing too hurriedly from a single protuberance. Take, for example, a well-developed organ of 'destructiveness'. If this happened to be accompanied both by a strong faculty of 'acquisitiveness' and a weak faculty of 'conscientiousness' then their owner might be led to commit a murder. If, on the other hand, the same faculty of 'destructiveness' happened to be accompanied by a strong faculty of 'benevolence' and strong 'conscientiousness' it might have quite the opposite effect. 'It might arrest the arm of the widow's oppressor' or encourage other equally good works. This was Gall's so-called 'doctrine of the combinations'. A good deal of nice judgement was evidently required of those who would exercise the arts of phrenology.

Opposite:
In the middle of the 19th century many hundreds of these ceramic heads were manufactured and sold

A bust showing the location of the mental 'faculties', according to Spurzheim, student and admirer of Dr. Gall, the founder of phrenology

A cartoon of William Pitt and King Gustavus IV Adolphus, consulting Dr. Gall incognito

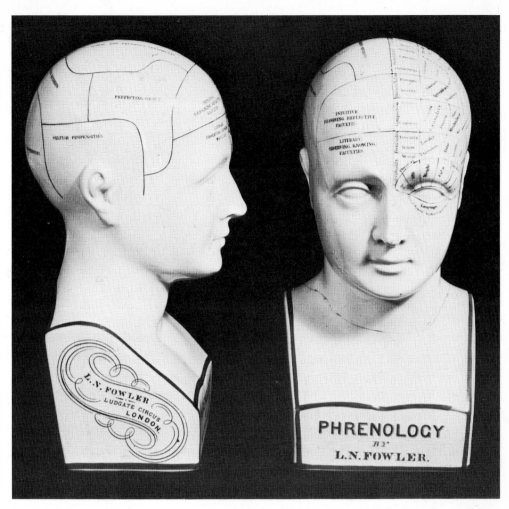

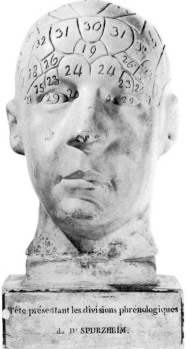

Tête présentant les divisions phrénologiques
du Dᵣ SPURZHEIM.

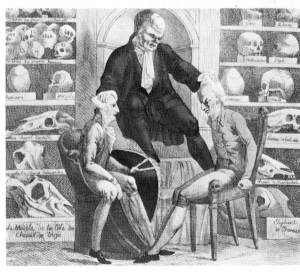

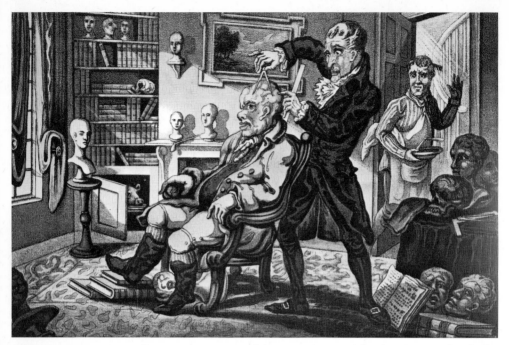

Cartoon of a craniological examination

It was because of its concern with the 'organs' of the brain that this strange pseudo-science became known for a time as 'organology'. Later it became 'cranioscopy' and finally 'phrenology'. It was destined to achieve great popularity in Gall's lifetime—and especially so following upon the eloquent propagandising of Spurzheim, one of his students and admirers. Spurzheim was largely responsible for the enormous popularity of phrenology throughout America and Europe. He lectured extensively and to large audiences both in the USA and in Europe. In 1832 he visited Boston to deliver a series of lectures and demonstrations to the Medical Faculty of Harvard where, it is said, 'the professors were in love with him'. He died, however, shortly after his arrival there, some said of exhaustion after being so enthusiastically welcomed and worked by his hosts. His funeral became something of a State occasion and the Boston Phrenological Society was hurriedly formed to his memory. For several years thereafter phrenology was taken very seriously indeed. Shortly after Spurzheim's death, George Combe, a Scottish lawyer, arrived in America to continue the master's teaching. He too captured the imagination of the intelligentsia of New England, at that time in the midst of the 'New England Renaissance'. The ideas of the phrenologists were soon to be spread far and wide throughout America, and eventually the rest of the world. Phrenology was, after all, an attractive, pleasingly democratic doctrine. The notion that all men were possessed of their own special talents, no doubt quite different from those of their neighbours, was a very persuasive one. Unlike the metaphysical and mystical pronouncements of many previous physiognomists and 'mental philosophers' of the time the phrenologists seemed to speak in a refreshingly rational, concrete, scientific way—and in those early days of the nineteenth century scientific ideas were becoming much in vogue.

Not surprisingly, there was considerable commercial exploitation of this seductive doctrine, particularly in America, where Messrs. Fowler and Wells (whose advertisement is illustrated) were only one of the many commercial organisations able to capitalise on the enormous growth of public interest in phrenology. 'Phrenological parlours' were opened in all the major cities. Lecture tours were eagerly attended and often over-subscribed. Endless series of publications were produced. *Phrenological Self-Instructors* were published, and all kinds of equipment and measuring devices were manufactured and enjoyed a ready sale, as did charts, pointers, labelled skulls, busts and casts of heads of famous men. As well as becoming an industry, however, phrenology became a popular entertainment. It was soon every man's ambition to have his 'bumps read' at the earliest opportunity—whether at a fairground or in the comfortable 'Phrenological Parlours' of the city. Long, impressive questionnaires and 'rating scales' were provided to be filled in either by experts in the parlour or, in later 'self-measurement' versions, by oneself at home. There was even a practice, for a time, of requiring an applicant for a job to bring his phrenological chart with him to his interview— duly certified by a phrenologist. The form would indicate whether each of the twenty-seven faculties was 'large, medium or small', and contained a full analysis of the candidate's suitability for the job. It might also contain a full explanation of the implications of the measurements for health, happiness and even success in love and marriage as well as in work. Some of the examination forms went so far

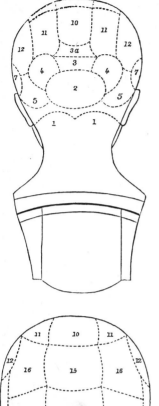

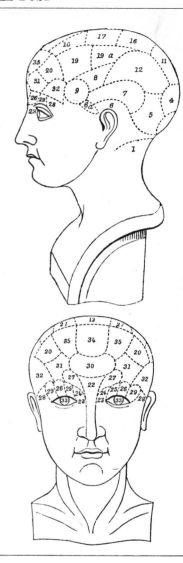

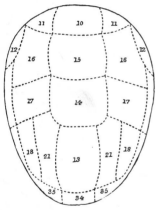

NAMES OF THE MENTAL FACULTIES, THE POSITIONS OF THE ORGANS OF WHICH ARE MARKED UPON THE BUST.

AFFECTIVE.

I. PROPENSITIES.

1. Amativeness, vol. i. p. 183
2. Philoprogenitiveness, 193
3. Concentrativeness, 211
3. a Inhabitiveness, ib.
4. Adhesiveness, . 237
5. Combativeness, . 243
6. Destructiveness, 255
6. a Alimentiveness, 277
7. Secretiveness, . 294
8. Acquisitiveness. . 311
9. Constructiveness, 326

II. SENTIMENTS.

10. Self-Esteem, vol. i. p. 341
11. Love of Approbation, 357
12. Cautiousness, . 369
13. Benevolence, . 382
14. Veneration, . 399
15. Firmness, . . 413
16. Conscientiousness, 418
17. Hope, . . . 443
18. Wonder, . . 449
19. Ideality, . . 469
19. a Unascertained, 477
20. Wit or Mirthfulness, 490
21. Imitation . . 511

INTELLECTUAL.

I. PERCEPTIVE.

22. Individuality,
    vol. ii. p. 28
23. Form, . 35
24. Size, . . . 41
25. Weight, . . 46
26. Colouring, . 53
27. Locality, . 72
28. Number, . . 83
29. Order, . . 90
30. Eventuality, . 92
31. Time, . . 104
32. Tune, . . 110
33. Language, 124

II. REFLECTIVE.

34. Comparison, vol. ii. p. 151
35. Causality, . . 163

MONGOLIAN. CAUCASIAN. MALAY.

OUTLINES

OF

PHRENOLOGY:

GIVING

THE FIRST PRINCIPLES OF THE SCIENCE,

AND THE

Definition of the Organs,

INCLUDING THEIR

USE, EXCESS, AND DEFICIENCY.

CONN. SUEDENING.

Know Thyself.

DR. GALL.

By FOWLER AND WELLS.

Phrenologists and Publishers,

308 BROADWAY,

NEW YORK.

RICAN. AM. INDIAN.

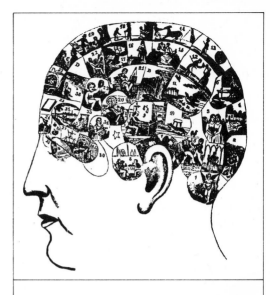

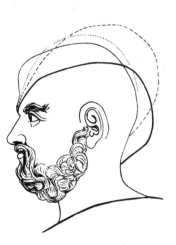

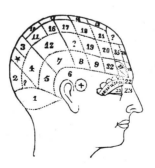
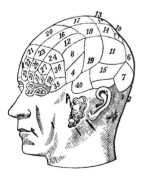

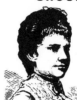

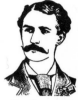

as to specify in detail the characteristics recommended for an 'ideal' marriage partner, including such features as hair and eye colour and complexion, as well as the recommended temperament for the spouse. It is easy to see how the commercial phrenologists prospered.

Phrenology was eventually attacked by churchmen, largely because of its radical, even atheistic, implications. One of the assertions of phrenological doctrine was that moral behaviour depended entirely on the body, upon the 'organ of reverence'; and this was, of course, for many, a quite unacceptable notion.

Meanwhile, in the middle of the nineteenth century, neurologists and anatomists were beginning to discover the true functions of the different parts of the brain. Broca, for example, in 1861, showed clearly that the region of the brain responsible for speech and language was not located behind the eyes, as Gall had declared and as thousands of Fowler's pot busts had so confidently proclaimed, but in a very different place: on the left temporal lobe of the brain, above the left ear.

Gall's whole 'doctrine of the skull' was, as we now realise, quite without foundation. It is now known that differences of shape and size of the skull have little or no bearing on mental powers or on character qualities. People with large heads are no more, and no less, intelligent than those with small heads. People with small heads, like Erasmus, may be very intelligent indeed. Nor does character depend in any known way upon the size or shape of the head.

During the century since Gall's death a great deal more has been learned about the functions of the different parts of the brain. Neurologists no longer believe that different features of personality are located in particular parts of the brain. On the contrary, personality factors, like so many other features of brain activity important in everyday life, such as reasoning, planning and solving problems, are functions of the brain *as a whole,* or at least of very large, overlapping segments of it. No part of the brain has yet been discovered which is responsible by itself for 'mirthfulness' or 'tune' or 'intuition' or any of the other single qualities which the phrenologists so confidently declared as having their corresponding 'bumps'.

And yet, although the phrenologists were certainly mistaken in their basic beliefs, their influence has not been entirely harmful. As Bakan has pointed out, they increased popular interest in behaviour and personality and this has had many useful consequences. One of the teachings of the phrenologists, for example, was that children's learning occurred by 'proper exercise of the muscles of the mind'. Gall and Spurzheim urged 'learning by doing', and opposed the use of repetitive drill and learning by rote. They also insisted that punishment had no part to play in learning. And they objected to a school curriculum based, as then tended to be the custom, entirely on the Classics. All of the mental faculties, they urged, must be given the opportunity for exercise, so that every young mind might reach its true, God-given potential. Phrenologists advocated physical training and a shortening of the school day so that children could play freely and explore the world in their own creative way: ideas which were indeed novel in their day. Children, they insisted, could, given the opportunity, learn a great deal from their environment. These ideas led to recommendations for the improvement and redesign of school curricula, which would now be regarded as eminently sensible and progressive. But it was not only in relation to children that their ideas were so advanced. The teachings of the phrenologists led also to a much more humane approach to the mentally-ill. Psychiatric patients, they urged, should not be isolated and condemned as wholly beyond help. Rather, the task should be to discover which of their faculties were still whole and healthy and capable of retraining. The phrenologists advocated also a more optimistic approach towards the treatment of criminals whose talents for good should be explored and encouraged. The first systematic approach to the education of blind deaf mutes was also inspired by phrenology. Laura Bridgeman, a girl who was blind, deaf and mute but whose head 'bumps' were judged propitious by a phrenologist, was taught successfully to speak—the first of many such cases to be helped. It is strange that such valuable work should have been based on such erroneous theoretical foundations. Psychologists owe a great deal to phrenologists in yet another way: for their emphasis on the importance of studying the *differences* between individuals.

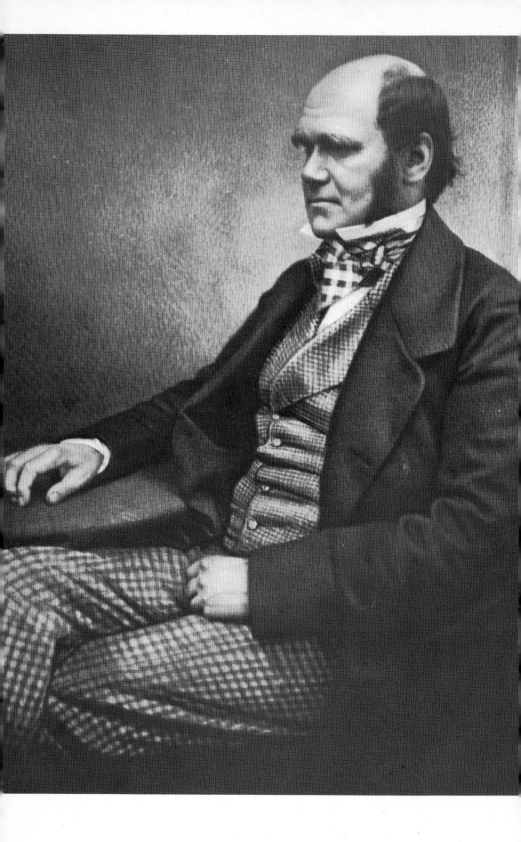

Hitherto it was human experience and behaviour in general which had been studied. The search was for 'laws' which applied to all mankind. The study of 'individual differences' has since been recognised as a most important and fundamental part of modern psychology. Nowadays, there is much more concern with questions of individual personality.

By the early years of the nineteenth century, the study of the face, like that of other natural phenomena, was rapidly becoming much more sophisticated. In 1806, Sir Charles Bell, in his *Anatomy and Philosophy of Expression*, made a brilliant analysis of the physical foundations, as well as the purposes, of facial movements. Thereafter, scientific, though not popular, interest in old-fashioned physiognomy declined, and new works on the face were concerned, by and large, with detailed physiological problems, such as Burgess's interesting work on *The Physiology or Mechanisms of Blushing* (1839), and papers like those of Bain, Herbert, Spencer and Piderit, which collected together valuable observations on expression.

And soon there was to come, in 1859, Darwin's great work *On the Origin of Species*, in which, among other things, he gave an account of facial communication throughout the animal kingdom—a more detailed work on which he published in 1872: *The Expression of the Emotions in Man and Animals*. Much of his scientific material for these books was collected during his famous voyage on HMS *Beagle*. And yet this journey very nearly did not take place. As Darwin later related in his *Autobiography*, the Captain of the 'Beagle' did not like the look of the scientist's face:

> Afterwards on becoming very intimate with the Captain, I heard that I had run a very narrow risk of being rejected on account of the shape of my nose! He was an ardent disciple of Lavater and was convinced that he could judge of a man's character by the outline of his features, and he doubted whether anyone with my nose could possess sufficient energy and determination for the voyage.

It would have been a strange irony of fate if Darwin had been prevented from undertaking this voyage by the very subject he was destined so brilliantly to advance. Fortunately, Darwin was allowed aboard and he made the voyage —in spite of the shape of his nose.

Guides to character?

The 'science' of phrenology almost prevented Darwin from making his historic voyage on HMS Beagle

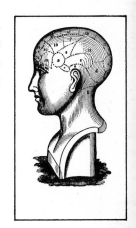

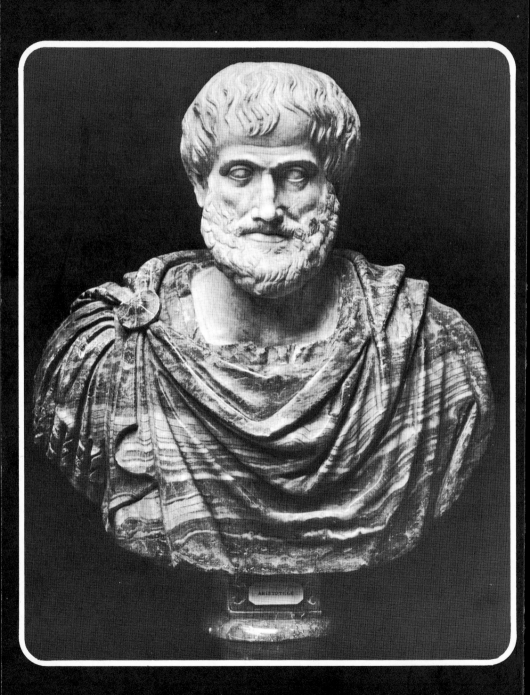

According to Aristotle, a high forehead was a mark of
intellect; large eyebrows were a sign of cowardice and
timidity; large ears, 'a tendency to irrelevant talk or chattering'. As we have seen, beliefs of this kind, that there is a
simple, direct relationship between facial feature and character, have always existed. Old textbooks of physiognomy are
full of advice on the important 'signs' to be found in the
face. It would be useful, therefore, to review some of this
advice in a little more detail and consider its validity in the
light of modern knowledge.

It was always the eyes, more than any other facial feature,
that particularly fascinated ancient writers. Paracelsus, the
mediaeval scholar, believed them to be by far the most
valuable of all the facial indicators.

Blackness of the eyes generally denotes health, a firm
mind, not wavering but courageous, true and honourable. Grey eyes generally denote deceit, instability and in-
decision. Short sight denotes an able projector, crafty and
intriguing in action.

The squinty or false-eyed who see on both sides, or over
and under, certainly denotes a deceitful crafty person,
not easily deceived, mistrustful and not to be trusted,
one who willingly avoids labour when he can, indulging
in idleness, play, usury and pilfering.

Small, deep sunken eyes are untrying and active in
wickedness. Large eyes denote a covetous greedy man
and especially when they are prominent.

The winking eye denotes an amorous disposition.

Red eyes signify courage and strength.

Bright eyes, slow of motion, bespeak the hero, great acts,
audacious, cheerful, one feared by his enemies.

For Lavater, too, the eyes were the most powerful of all
signals of character. Choleric men, for example, had eyes
which were 'more brown rather than blue.' 'Green eyes',
on the other hand, indicated 'ardour, fire and courage'.
'Clear blue eyes' accompanied a 'phlegmatic temperament'.

Eye colour has long been regarded as an indication of
character. In western folklore and literature blue eyes have
traditionally been associated with gentleness and goodness
and dark eyes with passion and sensuality. Even religious
significance has, in some countries, been attached to the

*Opposite Aristotle,
one of the earliest writers
on physiognomy, believed
a high forehead to be a
mark of intellect, and
large ears 'a tendency to
irrelevant talk or
chattering'*

colour of the eyes. Grey eyes, for example, like red beards, are anathema to orthodox Moslems, who take them to be a sign of sin, enmity and cowardice—possibly because the traditional enemies of Moslem peoples centuries ago were the Greeks, many of whom were grey-eyed and red-bearded.

Eyebrows, too, have been of great concern to physiognomists, both ancient and modern. The Arab philosopher and physician Avicenna believed that well-developed eyebrows were an unfailing indication of craftiness and guile. Lavater, on the other hand, believed they were a sign of strength of character and intellect:

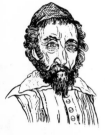

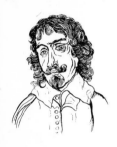

> Angular, strong, interrupted eyebrows ever denote fire and productive activity . . .
> I never yet saw a profound thinker, or a man of fortitude and prudence with weak high eyebrows.

But their position was equally important:

> The nearer the eyebrows are to the eyes the more earnest, deep and firm the character. The more remote from the eyes the more volatile, easily moved and less enterprising. Remote from each other, warm, open, quick [of] sensation. White eyebrows signify weakness, and dark brown, firmness. Eye-bones with defined, marked, easily-delineated firm arches I never saw but in noble and in great men. All the ideal antiques [Greek portrait busts] have these arches. . . .

Della Porta believed that

> strong brows show the power, the mightiness and the ferocity of the lion.

Thomas Hill, writing in the sixteenth century, declared that

> a brow developed in length indicates good sense and plenty of faculty for the sciences.

Lavater, however, disagreed with the old physiognomists as to the significance of eyebrows which met in the middle:

> Meeting eyebrows, held so beautiful by the Arabs and by the old physiognomists supposed to be the work of craft, I can neither believe to be beautiful nor characteristic of such a quality. Meeting eyebrows are to be found in the most honest and worthy countenances though it is true they give the face a gloomy appearance and perhaps denote trouble of mind and heart.

But after the eyes and brows, according to Lavater, it was

the forehead which most proclaimed the man.

I consider the peculiar delineation of the outline and position of the forehead . . . to be the most important of all the things presented to physiognomical observation. The longer the forehead, the more comprehension and the less activity. . . .

The more compressed the forehead the more compression, firmness and the less volatility in the man. Perfect perpendicularity, from the hair to the eyebrow, the want of understanding, but perfect perpendicularity gently arched at the top denotes excellent propensities of cold, tranquil, profound thinking. Perpendicular foreheads . . . which are small, wrinkly, short and shining are certain signs of weakness, little understanding, little imagination. Retreating foreheads in general denote superiority of imagination and acuteness.

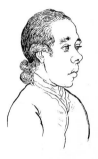

His views on the intellectual implications of the forehead, therefore, run counter to those of Aristotle—and indeed many other physiognomists, before and since his own time.

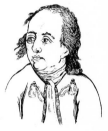

It is not altogether surprising that Lavater, who himself had a receding forehead, should value this especially highly as a mark of intellect. Aristotle, on the other hand, whose brow, from surviving sculpture, seems to have been vertical, predictably valued a high, straight brow. But we shall return to this important question of 'narcissistic choice' in a later chapter.

Lavater's interest in the face was much more than intellectual, however. He wrote with real passion of its beauty—captivated especially by the *rare* beauty of the nose:

I meet with thousands of beautiful eyes before one beautiful nose. Such a nose is worth more than a Kingdom; it is never found associated with an ugly face.

He described the perfect nose:

It should have a length equal to that of the forehead. At the top there should be a gentle indenting. The button or end of the nose should be neither hard nor fleshy. Viewed in profile the bottom of the nose should not have been more than one third of its length.

Still, beautiful or ugly, the nose seemed to him an unfailing guide to character:

a beautiful nose denotes an extraordinary character.

A selection of beliefs,
ancient and modern,
about facial detail
A   Aristotle
AV Avicenna
DP Della Porta
H   Hill
L   Lavater
P   Paracelsus
M   Modern students

Large ears/irrelevant talker, chatterer A
Small deep sunken eyes/wickedness P
Large eyes (prominent)/greedy P
Eye colour:
green/ardour, fire, courage L
blue/gentleness, goodness L
dark/passion, sensuality L
black/health, firmness, courage P
Well-developed eyebrows/craftiness and guile AV
„   „   „   /strength of character and
                              intellect L
Eyebrows close to eyes/earnest, deep, firm character L
Eyebrows distant from eyes/volatility L
Eyebrows widely separated/warm and open L
Firm-arched eye-bones/nobility and greatness L
Long brows/faculty for the sciences H
Angular, interrupted brows/mental productiveness DP
Meeting eyebrows/honesty, worthiness L
Long forehead (receding)/great intellect L
Perpendicular forehead/'want of understanding' L
„   „   /great intellect A
Arched nose/commanding, ruling, powerful L
Large nose/dominance, bossiness, arrogance M
Small nose/femininity, weakness, submissiveness,
    complacency M
Concave nose/forbearance, imagination L
Large mouth/extraversion M
Small mouth/introversion or meanness or slyness M
Firm lips/firm character L
Thin lips/coldness, love of order and precision L
Lips if tilted up at corners/affectation,
    pretension, vanity L
Projecting chin/'positive' character L
Indent in middle of chin/'cool understanding' L
Double chin/the epicure L

He conceded, however, that

there are indeed innumerable excellent men with defective
hollow noses but their worth lies not so much in character
as in forbearance, in suffering, in listening, learning and
in enjoying the beautiful influences of imagination.

Socrates, he noted, had the ugliest of noses, but was a great
man, full of gentleness and patience.

Furthermore:

Noses which are arched near the forehead, are capable of
command, they can rule, act, overcome . . . destroy. I
have never yet seen a nose with a broad back, whether
arched or rectilinear, that did not appertain to an extraordinary man. We may examine thousands of countenances, and numberless portraits of superior men before
we find such a one.

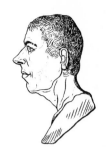

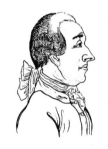

He cited Swift, Raynal, Caesar Borgia, Peter de Medici,
Caracci and Titian in support of his thesis.

For Leonardo da Vinci, too, the nose was the great
character-maker. 'Make comparisons!' he said, the nose is
the '*honastamentum faciei*': it provides the key to the character
of the whole face. It is also the prime aid in recalling the
face to memory.

But the shape of the nose has always been a deep concern
of physiognomists, professional and amateur. Some strange
beliefs have been held about its racial and even religious
significance. Many people have believed, for example, that
there is a 'typically Jewish' nose—by which they usually
mean a convex, arched nose, hooked at the tip. Yet a
research study made in New York in 1952, in which 2,836
male and 1,284 female Jews were examined, revealed that
57% of the males had flat noses, 14% concave, 6.4% flared
and only about one fifth, 22.3%, convex. Very similar
results were obtained by Liejnec in Poland. His findings, too,
show quite clearly that there is no such thing as a 'characteristically Jewish' nose. A high-arched nose does, however,
seem to occur quite frequently among American Indians
and some Armenian peoples.

As for character implications of the *chin*, Lavater was in
no doubt whatsoever:

I am, from numerous experiments, convinced that the
projecting chin ever denotes something positive, and the

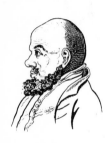

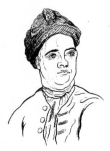

retreating something negative. The presence or absence of strength in man is often signified by the chin. I have never seen sharp indentings in the middle of the chin but in men of cool understanding unless when something evidently contradictory appeared in the countenance. The soft fat double-chin generally points out the epicure; and the angular chin is seldom found but in discreet, well-disposed, firm men. Flatness of chin speaks the cold and dry: smallness, fear: and roundness with a dimple, benevolence.

Such enviable certainty!

The mouth itself has often excited the imagination not only of physiognomists but of philosophers and poets too. The German philosopher Herder once declared:

It is from the mouth that the voice issues, interpreter of the heart and of the soul, expression of feeling, of friendship and of the purest enthusiasm. The upper lip translates the inclinations, the appetites, the disquietude of love; pride and passion contract it, cunning accentuates it; goodness of heart reflects it; debauchery enervates and debases it, love and the passions incarnate themselves there with an inexpressible charm.

Lavater was even more moved:

This part of the body is so sacred to me that I scarcely dare speak of it. What a subject of admiration! The mouth is the interpreter and organ of the mind and of the heart. In repose, as in the infinite variety of its movements, it unites a world of characters. It is eloquent, even in its silence.

Tommaseo, in his *Moral Thoughts* even went so far as to express the view that the mouth was nothing less than 'the repository of the soul'. Lavater, again, echoed something of this mystical view in his description of the mouth of a woman beloved:

The woman whose eyes have awakened our love inspires us with enthusiasm, exalts us, throws us into intellectual ecstasy; but she whose mouth fascinates us twines us round, binds us, belongs to us already, at least in the irresponsible world of desires. The eye is the azure heaven to which none may attain; the mouth is the earth with its perfumes, its ardours, and the profound sensuality of its points.

And yet, as Lavater explained, the mouth of even an
ordinary mortal displays his merits and demerits for all to
see:

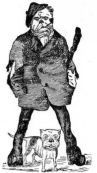

> As are the lips so is the character. Firm lips, firm character;
> weak lips, weak and wavering character. Well-defined,
> large and proportionate lips, the middle line of which is
> equally serpentine on both sides, and easy to be drawn,
> though they may denote an inclination to pleasure, are
> never seen in a bad, mean, common, false crouching,
> vicious countenance. A lipless mouth, resembling a single
> line, denotes coldness, industry, a love of order, precision,
> housewifery; and if it be drawn upwards at the two ends
> affectation, pretension, vanity, and . . . malice. Very
> fleshy lips must ever contend with sensuality and indo-
> lance; the cut-through, sharp-drawn lip with anxiety
> and avarice.

A Real Bully.

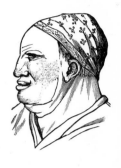

Lavater's *Essays on Physiognomy* are full of attractive, thoughtful and sometimes amusing conclusions such as these. His
overriding passion for the welfare of his fellow men, his
devout belief in man's basic goodness—and his deep concern that man should live in harmony with man—led him
with prodigious energy to seek out and describe every
single minute detail which might help us all the better to
understand ourselves and each other.

The great excitement generated by Lavater's writings,
both in Europe and America, encouraged many imitators,
and during the early years of the nineteenth century his
work was much plagiarized. Unfortunately many of his
imitators had neither Lavater's ability, his sensitivity, nor
his genuine concern for his fellow men. Many, too, were
quite overcome with enthusiasm for their subject. Consider
for example the account given by Simms in 1888 of 'that
wonderful quality of *elevativeness*'—the signs of which were
so clearly to be seen in the face.

'Elevativeness', he explained,

> is that nobleness, loftiness and exaltation of mind which
> will ever carry you up from the base and the mercenary
> up towards the elevated and magnanimous.

Given such a quality,

> you will ever desire to raise your body, mount a horse,

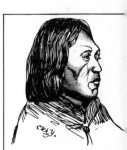

Elevativeness small
Flat Head Indian
of Puget Sound.

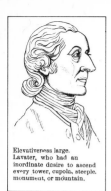

climb trees, ascend church steeples, rise in a balloon and hope to go up, when done with this earthly form.

The unmistakable and unfailing facial sign of elevativeness, as Simms declared, was

a nose that stands well out and up at the point.

Another characteristic described by Simms as visible in the face was one which most of us no doubt would wish to avoid. He called it the quality of '*retaliativeness*':

Rigorous, implacable and unforgiving, you scarcely ever relent. Always able and ready to retort in a vindictive manner, you naturally seek revenge for imaginary or real injuries.

The 'sign of retaliativeness', according to Simms,

is a hollow in the centre of the forehead. The elephant is an example of such a revengeful character; and the hippopotamus and rhinoceros are exceedingly retaliative. Horses with this deep indent in the forehead should never be trusted.

In another popular book of the late nineteenth century, *Faces We Meet and How to Read Them*, R. B. D. Wells offered the following advice to shopkeepers:

Some ladies are hard to please in the selection of a pattern for a new dress. Shopkeepers would save themselves a deal of trouble, and suit their customers better, if they were to bear in mind that as a general rule, *ladies with long features prefer a long pattern* while those with round and small features prefer a small and rounded pattern.

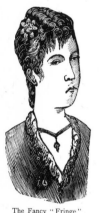

The Fancy "Fringe" —accompanying a proud and vain disposition— more show than substance.

It would be unfair however, to condemn a whole tradition because of the excesses of its less able exponents. There is and always has been a strong human drive towards comprehension and understanding of all the things around us, and —as Lavater realised and was so anxious to promote— nowhere has this been more evident than in the need for an understanding of the people we meet, the people with whom we daily have to deal. Perhaps this explains the permanent popularity, the timeless, universal appeal, of physiognomy. We must *know* our fellow men, we must feel we understand them.

Opposite *A study of eight grotesque heads by Leonardo da Vinci*

The particular aspects we look for in the face of others will clearly vary according to our different needs, interests, desires, past experiences. An aged person will generally

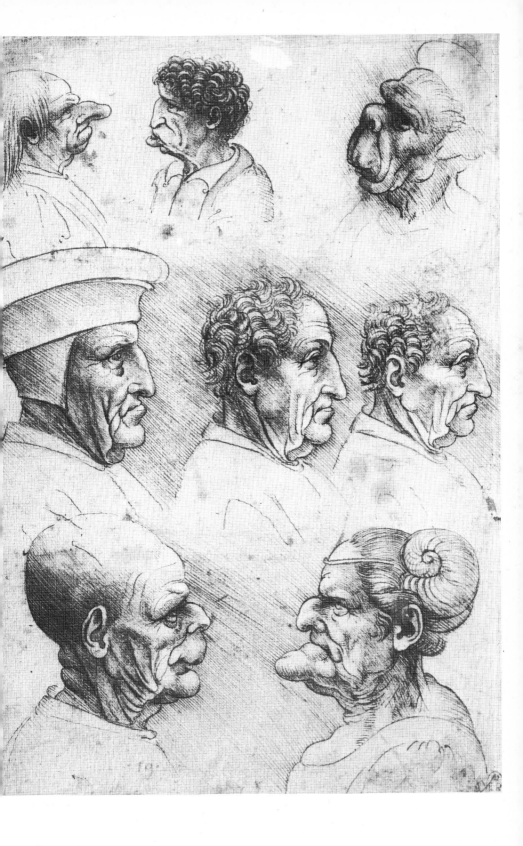

The characteristics which people see in the faces of others often tell us more about the person who is looking at the face than about the person being viewed. This discovery has been put to good use in the Liggett Faces Test, a test which has been deliberately designed to reveal the viewer's personality

The Faces Test, part of which is shown here, contains deliberately vague and indistinct portraits—almost as vague as inkblots. The person being tested is asked to offer his opinions about the probable personality of the 'people' depicted. The answers given are extremely varied. But a pattern has emerged. Introverts react quite differently from extroverts and answers given by normal healthy people are different from those given by people who are suffering from psychiatric illness. Research with 782 people (470 psychiatric patients, 312 normal people) has shown that the kind of answers given can provide the psychologist with a reliable indicator of the personality of the individual taking the test. See specimen answers on right—
P Psychiatric patients
N Normal people

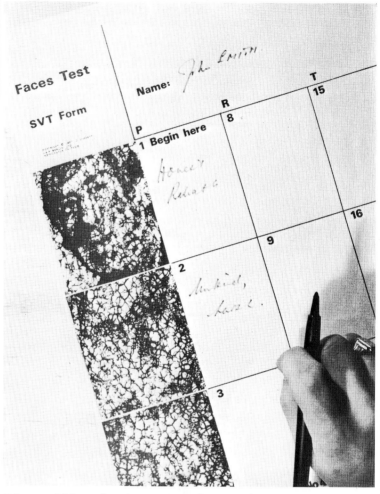

'He would be a dominant sort of person' P 28% N 17%
'He would be inquisitive' P 23% N 2%
'He would be married' P 18% N 4%
'He would be a helpful person' P 19% N 32%
'He would be about ... years old' P 26% N 41%
'He would be a happy, jolly person' P 21% N 39%

These results suggest that the qualities perceived in these ink-blot faces are certainly influenced by the personality of the individual looking at them. The interesting question now arises as to whether the same is true with faces in real life. It is tempting to speculate that when character judgements are made from real faces, the character qualities which are seen may, like beauty, originate in the eye and mind of the beholder.

have interests and needs different from those of a teenager. Whereas the older person will crave helpfulness and generosity the youngster will seek excitement and activity. So it is natural that the older person will look for signs of kindness and gentleness much more than signs of sexual interest; a cheat will look for gullibility; the chairman of an Officer Selection Board will look for power and decisiveness. But our interest in and preoccupations about other people vary widely not only from person to person but also from group to group and age to age. Indeed, it is this very diversity of approach that we all display to the world of people which helps make us the unique personalities we are.

As the writer's own research with his 'Faces Test' has shown, a great deal can be learnt about a person from the categories he uses in describing the faces of others. When asked to describe the very vague 'faces' in the Test in their own words, psychiatric patients, for example, use very different categories from those employed by normal, healthy people.

The important question which must eventually be answered is whether the signs and signals we believe we can see in people's faces have any utility as indicators of intellect and character. Many men have clearly thought so—many of them wise, brilliant and sensitive men—and there are countless people today who firmly believe the face and its features to be one of the best and most powerful guides to character. A survey of University students by the writer showed that such beliefs may be held with surprising tenacity.

The face was considered by the majority of these students to be a helpful guide to personality—and the eyes and mouth, especially so. About half of them considered the chin and jaw important guides. Scepticism was rare: rather less than ten per cent of all those who answered the questionnaire were prepared to say that 'there were no important facial guides to character'. A substantial number, on the contrary, believed the face to be a valuable guide to social class. The size of the mouth was generally felt to be important: a *large mouth* indicating extraversion, a *small mouth* introversion. A *large nose* indicated dominance, bossiness and arrogance—surprisingly few students came to the

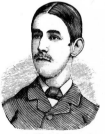

An Effeminate Man.

traditional physiognomist's conclusion of 'sexual vigour'. A *small nose,* on the other hand, was widely believed to indicate femininity, weakness and submissiveness.

Here then we have recent evidence of firm conviction about the correlation of character and the face. But how can we confirm that such conviction is justified—that there really are, in truth, consistent relationships between personality and facial features? We may respect Lavater's assertions as the opinions of an extremely active and astute observer of human nature based on the great numbers of men he studied —but we can hardly accept his statements as scientific evidence. It is clear that to achieve any kind of certainty we shall need two sorts of information: first, precise and un-ambiguous descriptions of facial characteristics—a system of classification of noses, eyes and brows about which there can be no argument—and secondly, we shall need equally precise and unambiguous descriptions and measurements of qualities of personality and character. Now it is with the second of these requirements, of course, that we run into particular difficulty: even the most straightforward character qualities are hard to define, let alone measure. Consider, for example, the quality of 'honesty'. In an attempt to study this Hartshorne and May spent a great deal of time with children during their *Character Education Enquiry.* They found that children are often scrupulously honest in some situations but not in others. Honesty is clearly not a quality that can be measured and transformed into a score which can then be assigned as a permanent grading to a child. And if there are such problems with apparently simple variables like honesty how are we to deal with many of the other more subtle qualities—greed, malice, altruism— about which the physiognomists had so much to say?

Though this is our main problem—the accurate specifica-tion and measurement of the psychological qualities of character and personality—we are still not without diffi-culties on the other, the purely *physical* side, of the equation. Seemingly obvious facial features are not nearly as easy to describe and categorise as one might suppose. The great French ethnologist Topinard found himself in great difficulty classifying such a straightforward feature as the nose. Leonardo da Vinci gave up the attempt after describing ten major types of nose and several more sub-types. Are we then likely to succeed in producing a convincing categorisation of 'arched brows' or 'strong chins'—a firm enough foundation on which to build?

The problem of the recording and analysis of facial features and facial patterns will eventually have to be solved by much more sophisticated techniques than we now possess. The description and measurement of character and temperament will probably best be made by the use of such mathematical methods as 'factor analysis' now being so successfully developed by Cattell and Eysenck. It is fortunate that, for the first time in history, the instrument needed to undertake the prodigious mathematical calculations needed for these new techniques has become available in the computer. But we shall have to be patient, and await the verdict of these new computational techniques in order to declare whether there is, in truth, any relationship, causal or otherwise, between face and personality.

Certainly, there are few professional psychologists today who believe that there is any correlation between our personality and facial features. All the evidence, on the contrary, suggests that we are what we are because of our 'nature'—our inherited predispositions—on the one hand, and our 'nurture'—our environment and education—on the other. And of these, it is probably nurture rather than nature which is the more important.

Paradoxically, however, there is a sense in which it *does not matter* whether there are any real causal relationships between personality and facial features. What matters most is that people sincerely believe that such relationships exist, and that such beliefs are commonly and widely held. Because if this is the case people will *act* as if such relationships exist—and a number of important consequences will necessarily follow.

If, for example, we are seen to possess narrowly-spaced eyes, people may very well treat us as though we were dishonest. If our brow is low they may regard us as unintelligent—and they may act towards us accordingly. Unjust though this process is, other people's behaviour, continuing over months and years, cannot fail to leave its mark on our personality. On the other hand, of course, the very same processes can act to our advantage: we may be helped—perhaps just by the colour of our eyes. A very popular and widely held stereotype, for example, is that blue eyes indicate gentleness and integrity. A girl with 'angelic' blue eyes might therefore very well receive far more credit than she deserves. It is by no means unreasonable to suppose that such a girl would acquire, over the years, an increasingly benign attitude to a world so full of people who regard her as possessed of such beautiful angelic qualities. As a result, she can hardly fail to become all the more pleasant, all the more cheerful—her whole personality might very well be changed for the better—and the generalisation about girls with blue eyes only strengthened all the more.

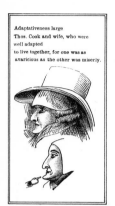

Adaptativeness large
Thos. Cook and wife, who were well adapted
to live together, for one was as avaricious as the other was miserly.

At the same time there is another, quite different way in which facial features and personality may come to be related. During the course of our lifetime a feature of our own we consider to be faulty or ugly may assume an undue importance in our mind—and our personality development be much inhibited in consequence. It is easy enough to see how the hideous nose of Rostand's Cyrano de Bergerac rendered him impotent to express his feelings directly to the woman he loved. Yet much lesser blemishes than this may inhibit us. They may even change our behaviour so that people begin to react to us in a quite different way. If we are convinced, for example, that our eyes are too narrow and deep-set—and if we are also convinced that this indicates a mean and shifty nature—we will perhaps begin to be less inclined to look people straight in the eye—and so may very well begin to acquire all the 'marks' of meanness and shiftiness. The tragedy is that in so many cases of this kind the troubling feature is objectively not nearly so bad nor so extreme as we fear. Indeed it may not even exist. Facial 'faults' are often more imagined than real. Yet, as we saw in the chapter on cosmetic surgery, such imagined defects can induce profound depression and cause much distress. This is the main and most serious danger of the pseudoscience of physiognomy. Not only can it seriously affect those who, by the merest chance of genetics, happen to possess a feature vulnerable to one or other of physiognomy's hard and fast rules; it can also badly upset those who merely *imagine* they possess any such feature. It is altogether wrong that such unhappiness should be generated by mere 'rules' which are themselves quite unsubstantiated and which, in all probability, are quite untrue.

It is pleasing to discover in this connection that the arch physiognomist, Lavater himself—unlike many of his predecessors and successors—steadfastly refused to discuss the facial characteristics of evil men. He had much more to say about the signs of goodness—and in this was being no less than true to his principles, to the objectives he declared even in the title of his great work: *Essays on Physiognomy: designed to promote the love of mankind.*

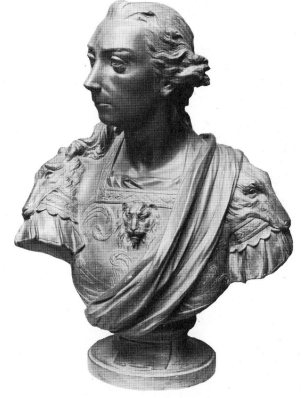

According to the rules of some of the old physiognomists, General Wolfe should have had neither courage (receding chin) nor intellect (receding forehead). He was, in fact, in his lifetime renowned for both of these qualities. Portrait sculpture by Joseph Wilton

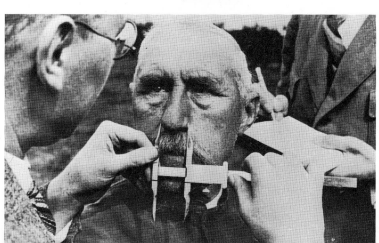

Racial determination in Nazi Germany: a modern example of the abuses which may follow in the wake of a pseudo-science such as physiognomy

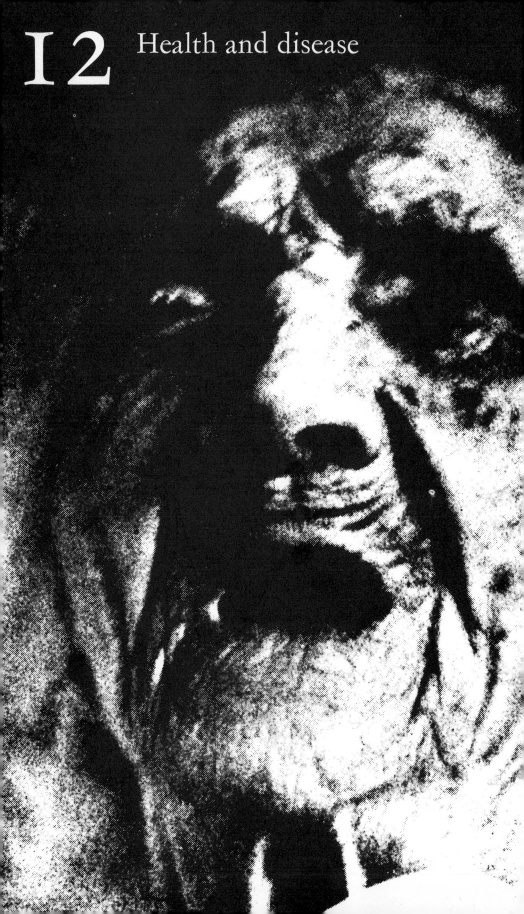

Hippocrates, 'the father of medicine', described as long ago as 400 BC the most fateful face of all, the *facies hippocratica* —the face of those about to die:

> Nose sharp, eyes hollow, temples shrunken, ears cold and contracted with their lobes turned outwards, the skin about the face hard and tense, the colour of the face being yellow or dark.

And there were many other ancient writers on the facial signs of illness—like Leomnius, Emilus, Campolongus— as well as, in more recent times, Wolff and Hoffmann. An important work was written on the subject in 1784 by Samuel Quelmalz: *De Prosoposcopia Medica*.

Remarkably, Lavater, who was himself the son of a physician, wrote very little about illness—only four pages 'On the condition of Health and Disease' in Volume III chapter iii of his *Essays on Physiognomy*. Though his comments were brief they were well in accord with later medical observations. He had this to say about the medical significance of the general appearance of the face:

> The observing mind examines the physiognomy of the sick, the signs of which extend over the whole body; but the progress and change of the disease is principally to be found in the countenance and its parts.

The furrows, corrugations and lines of the face have long been regarded as valuable diagnostic signs. In 1820 Nicholas Jadelot described and classified the facial lines and discussed their diagnostic significance. A pronounced *oculozygomatic* line on a child's face indicated, he believed, a brain or nerve disease. In adults, on the other hand, it indicated disease of the sexual organs 'or even excessive masturbation'. An exaggerated *nasalis* line (from the nostril to the mouth) indicated disease of the intestines or of the stomach. A pronounced *labialis* line (from the corner of the mouth) suggested pain or difficulty in breathing, and a prominent *collateralis nasi* line (down from the nose, outside the *labialis* line) disease of the viscera of the thorax or abdomen. Predictably, most modern physicians are disinclined to accept Jadelot's rather oversimplified conclusions. Thomas Spencer Wells, the renowned nineteenth-century gynaecologist, however, described another important facial sign; the drawn, pinched, anxious face of women with ovarian

Opposite:
The most fateful face of all: 'facies hippocratica', the face of those about to die

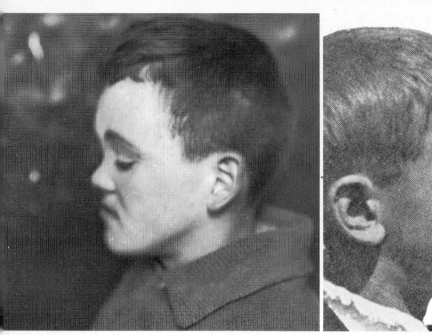

disease. Though we should perhaps note that Lavater had already declared many years previously:

In the *furor uterinus* the least observant can read the disease in the face.

James Lind, the naval surgeon of the eighteenth century, who achieved lasting fame by conquering scurvy with lime-juice, described the facial signs heralding that disease:

There is a change of colour of the face from the natural and usual look, to a pale and bloated complexion. The blood vessels of the lips and eyes take on a greenish cast.

The complexion of sailors affected with scurvy first became, as he explained, pale and yellowish, and later, as the disease progressed, darker and more livid. In the nineteenth century Sir Jonathan Hutchinson described the characteristics of the face in congenital syphilis: prominent frontal bosses to the skull and a depressed nasal bridge, later to become known as the 'saddle nose' of syphilis. Another nasal sign is well known: the florid red nose popularly associated with an excess of alcohol, but which may equally well be caused by heredity or by irritation of some kind (by freezing for example). The swollen bluish nose of cirrhosis of the liver due to alcoholic excess is still sometimes seen. The French physician Pierre Marie was the first to describe, in 1896, the large, coarse, elongated features,

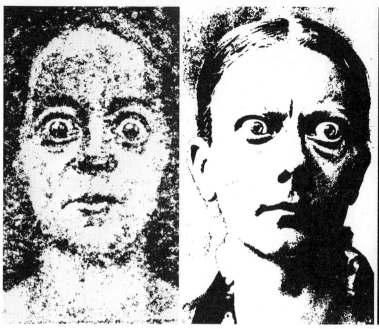

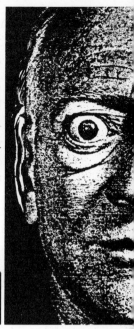

the swollen nose and prominent projecting lower jaw, which occur in *acromegaly* or gigantism, a condition caused by overactivity of the pituitary gland. In another glandular condition, Cushing's syndrome, the face sometimes develops a strangely 'moon-like' appearance.

Karl von Basedow, in the middle of the last century, described the face of exophthalmic goitre. This disease, caused by iodine deficiency, produces a wide-eyed stare and protruding eyes, and the thickened 'Derbyshire neck'. Another glandular disease which alters the facial appearance is Simmond's disease, a disorder of the pituitary and adrenal glands, which produces white and balding hair, and bodily wasting and weakness.

Over the last two centuries, a considerable number of facial signs of physical illnesses have become recognised and widely accepted. The early stages of typhoid fever, for example, are recognisable by a 'wild and bewildered' expression; the face is often dark and flushed. In heart disease the eyes often have a wide, staring appearance, the mouth is tense, and the whole face seems slightly shrunken. In yellow fever the face has a characteristic colouring, and in certain fevers in children the skin around the mouth becomes unusually pale. The yellow face of jaundice, too, is easily recognised. Another face once well known to

The wildly staring eyes of exophthalmic goitre, a condition associated with overactivity of the thyroid gland

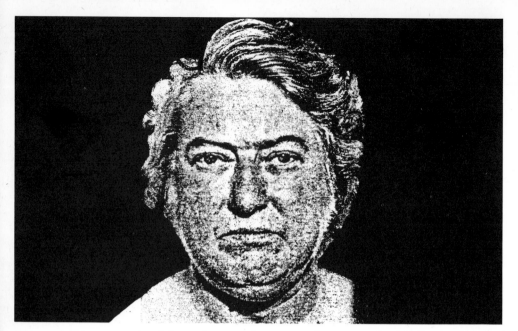

physicians, but rarely seen today, was the *'facies amabilis'* of tuberculosis. Here the eyes were lustrous, with bluish whites, the brow heavy, and the face immobile.

Changes in and around the eyes may provide important neurological signs. Unequal 'Argyll-Robertson' pupils, for example, are well known indicators of neurological damage. Sometimes the involvement of particular nerves can be recognised from facial signs: the onset of a squint or strabismus, for instance may signify malfunction in the fourth or sixth cranial nerves. Drooping eyelids or ptosis may indicate weakness in the third cranial nerve. In Bell's palsy there is abnormal relaxation in the whole of one side of the face due to paralysis of the seventh or 'facial nerve'.

Emil Kraepelin, who became famous for his revolutionary new ideas on the classification of mental illnesses, was convinced that there was a relationship between body-build and disease. He proposed the important concept of 'dia-thesis', which he considered to be 'an innate constitutional predisposition to a disease or a group of diseases.' The face, he believed, was one of the most important outward signs of the patient's diathesis. But this is in fact an old idea, dating back at least to the times of Hippocrates and Galen who had described the bodily and facial characteristics of 'apoplectic types' and 'consumptive types' and even 'gall-bladder

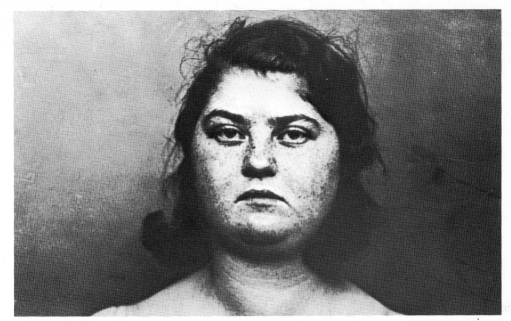

Above & opposite:
*The 'moon-like' face of
Cushing's disease,
another disorder in
which there is glandular
disturbance*

types'. Dr. Draper of Johns Hopkins University has recently produced striking evidence that susceptibility to certain diseases does indeed seem to be associated with particular facial proportions. He has found that tuberculosis, gall bladder disease, gastric ulcers and hypertension each have their own particular facial shapes and proportions. Draper observed that sufferers from the two very different diseases of pernicious anaemia and acromegaly tended to have the same facial proportions though different facial sizes, the face in anaemia being very much smaller.

A British psychiatrist once advanced the interesting view that in most forms of mental illness emotional expression is limited to the lower part of the face. It is true that many mental hospital patients seem to wear an immobile, permanently corrugated brow, but there are actually just as many who do not. The psychiatrist Ernst Kretschmer was impressed during his work in mental hospitals with the relationship between mental illness and the shape of the face. The tall, thin, hungry-looking patient, whom he described as 'asthenic', and who was, he believed, so often the sufferer from schizophrenic illness, was very likely, he decided, to have 'an egg-shaped face'. The profile would be sharp and angular, and there would often be a characteristic hair-line and hair distribution, giving the impression that

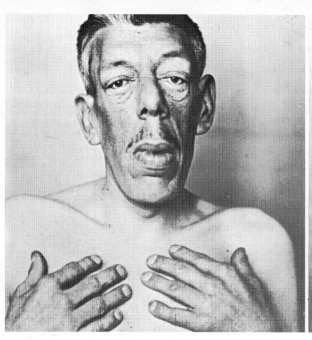
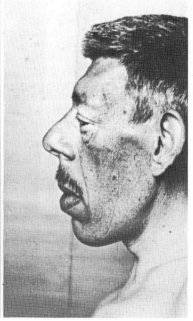

the patient was 'wearing a fur cap'. Kretschmer also described a quite different group of altogether broader, stronger-looking psychiatric patients. These were the ones likely to be suffering from 'affective' disorders such as depression or 'melancholia'. Here the facial form was 'likely to be shield-like'. The face would be broader and fuller and its outlines softer than those of the angular schizoid patient. Kretschmer noticed, too, that patients with affective illnesses commonly became bald at a comparatively early age. A more recent writer, C. W. Burr, has described the face of the melancholic in more detail:

> the lower jaw falls with or without a parting of the lips, making the face look long. Perpendicular wrinkles appear between the eyes, reach high up on the forehead and are crossed by horizontal ones. The opening between the eyelids is almost triangular. The corners of the mouth are drawn down, the under lip thrust forward.

It is the permanence of this expression, week in, week out, which is so characteristic of the melancholic. Nothing changes the expression, not even a sudden unexpected visit from a loved one, or news of an inherited fortune, or any other pleasant event. It is now realised by psychiatrists that on the rare occasions when facial changes in a melancholic do occur—furtive glances, perhaps, or a 'wandering'

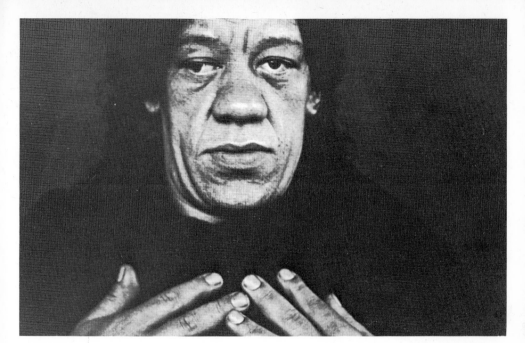

expression—they may provide useful signals to the nursing staff and may indicate the prelude to a suicidal attempt. But there are many modern psychiatrists who are by no means convinced that Kretschmer's ideas about the relationship between bodily and facial form and illness are at all helpful in the diagnosis of individual cases: there seem to be far too many exceptions to Kretschmer's general rules.

It is fair to say, in fact, that modern psychiatrists and physicians are rarely prepared to commit themselves to a diagnosis on the basis of a single sign—and certainly not a single facial sign. Indeed, nowadays there is no need for them to do so with such sophisticated diagnostic aids as X-rays, biochemical and bacteriological techniques, and a whole armoury of psychological diagnostic test methods which have proved so valuable in psychiatry. The process of decision for most physicians today is, in fact, an extraordinarily complex one, based on the skilled integration of many different signs perceived and symptoms reported, over perhaps a considerable period of time, and aided by much highly technical external information. From the medical point of view, therefore, the face is to be regarded as but one sign among many.

Above & opposite: The coarse features of Acromegaly, a condition associated with over-activity of the pituitary gland

13 Occupational faces

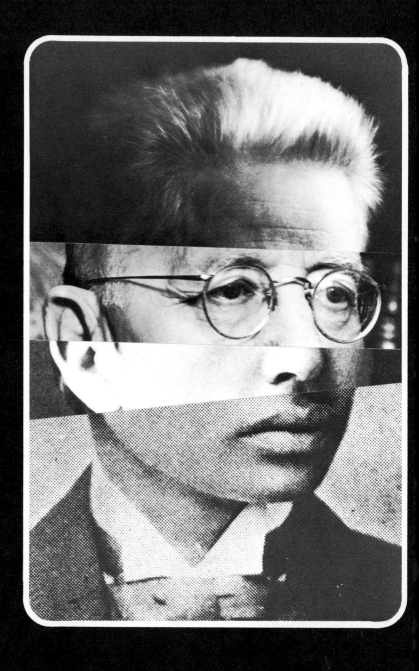

There are many people who believe that the stresses and strains of life show clearly in the face; that those who have led a happy life will have a smooth unruffled countenance, and those who have suffered deprivation and hardship will declare it in their wrinkles and furrows. It is tempting to believe that a harsh working environment will necessarily leave its marks on the face—that sailors and farmers, for example, will necessarily have a ruddy face and a tanned skin. But there are a number of writers, like the Italian physiognomist Paolo Mantegazza, who have gone a good deal further than this and declared that a man's profession invariably leaves its characteristic marks on his face—however gentle and benign his physical conditions of work. Prolonged maintenance of particular facial postures and particular habits of thought and attitude must, they say, be expected to leave their indelible marks on the face. Mantegazza declared, for example, that he could recognise carpenters 'in the midst of all other workmen who fashion and transform matter . . . their habit of planing, piercing, sawing, drawing lines, of seeing symmetry in the woods, gives a peculiar character to the muscles of the face—which becomes permanent.' He also believed that he could 'easily recognise the pharmacist among a host of other men.' This face, he declared, is 'associated with the gravity of the magician who reigns over prejudices, fears and mysteries.' The physician has something of this aspect, too, but usually, in addition, the 'stereotyped seriousness of the man who neither can nor will laugh in the midst of the suffering which he has constantly before his eyes.'

This belief in 'professional faces' is a popular one, and we should try to examine its validity. The specific thesis that prolonged expressions bring about permanent changes in the face deserves serious consideration if only because it has been proposed by so many eminent physiologists. It was many times asserted by the physiologists of expression of the nineteenth century, from Sir Charles Bell onwards, that constant use of certain muscle groups necessarily brings about structural changes in the facial tissue and that muscles which are not used become sluggish and, through lack of exercise, respond less readily. It must be said, however, that no substantial experimental or even observa-

Opposite *Composite photograph made up from portraits of Gandhi, Jensen, Chekhov, and Nielsen*

tional evidence has ever been adduced in support of this idea. It is difficult to imagine how such evidence could ever be obtained until entirely new and much more sophisticated methods are discovered for recording and describing facial patterns.

But even if we were to allow that a man's professional expressions might leave their mark on his countenance we would still need to enquire whether all men of a particular profession necessarily and habitually employ *similar* facial expressions. Are there, in fact, 'standard' professional postures? Is there, for example, a standard clerical expression? Or a standard facial posture for a family doctor? Only if this is shown to be the case can there be any sense in attempting to infer a man's profession from his face. We must, at least, consider the possibility that such postures exist—that they might even constitute social imperatives: that the parson in the proper execution of his duties might be expected to maintain a serious, far-sighted, sincere air, or that the General or Field-Marshal should show a keen-eyed firmness of countenance which will carry conviction in those he is required to command. No doubt there are professions where the ability to 'project' in this way might be considered an essential prerequisite of success: the face must fit the job. And if this is the case then it follows that the selection process itself will—if the selectors are competent—inevitably tend to perpetuate the stereotype. Commando officers must look like Commando officers. But there is also another selection process at work. For those men fortunate enough to be able to select their vocation, the choice of profession is often conditioned by successes and failures in early life and adolescence. These successes, on the games field and elsewhere, may well have a great deal to do with accidents of a man's physique and appearance. So it is evident that both institutionalised and personal selective processes are at work, and both may very well lead to the same stereotyped end-product. For several reasons, therefore, we should expect to find something approaching a 'military face' in the professional soldier. But can we seriously expect this to be the case in all professions?

Ernst Kretschmer, whose ideas on the face in mental illness we have already discussed, made an important and detailed study in his *Geniale Menschen* of the physique and faces of men of genius. He considered many examples over the centuries of poets and authors, artists, scholars, scientists and 'leaders and heroes' of great ability. He found ample confirmation of his basic belief that there was a relationship between face and character—that shy, retiring, contemplative individuals generally had the 'asthenic' physique, with angular, thin and perhaps drawn faces, and that sociable, extraverted and active people generally had features which were full, with softly rounded contours. Many of the great scientists of the past—such as Copernicus, Kepler, Liebnitz, Newton, and Faraday—were, as he expected, after consulting records of their personalities and interests, men with thin, angular faces. Indeed, he could find few examples of scientists who were of the ample, comfortable physique with rounded facial form, which he described as 'pyknic', and was led to the startling conclusion that most of the scientists of former times were lean asthenics with angular faces. The same was true of theologians, philosophers and jurists; Erasmus, Spinoza and Kant were, he found, all of the thin, 'asthenic' form, in both face and body. On the other hand, and as he had predicted from a knowledge of their personalities and activities, Kretschmer found that revolutionaries and men of action like Mirabeau and Luther were of variable cycloid disposition, and consequently of ample 'pyknic' physical form and rounded facial features. Among artists he discovered examples of both facial types—but again there was often a correspondence of physique and personality and style. The lusty, vigorous, extraverted style of Frans Hals was matched by his pyknic physique and features. Michelangelo, on the other hand, 'master of classic beauty and pathos', was, predictably, fine of feature and angular in physique.

Sir Francis Galton, the great English nineteenth-century eugenicist and pioneer student of 'individual differences', pursued this problem with characteristic energy. His predictably ingenious method of enquiry was to produce a 'face-mix'—a sort of 'average face' compounded of many separate individual portraits of men in a particular profession. He did this by a photographic method, superimposing many negatives in turn on the same sheet of photographic printing paper. His attractive and persuasively simple argument was that 'truly characteristic' features—big ears, for example, which occurred often in a collection of many negatives—would show clearly in the final print by the repeated exposures, whereas very variable features would print too faintly and would be lost: a large and a small mouth, for example, would fail to reinforce each other and would produce simply a blur in the final print. He assembled such composite pictures of many different social groups—criminals among them. He hoped that 'criminal features'—perhaps peculiarly shaped foreheads or elongated ears—would, by frequent repetition, become clear in his composite photographs. His expectation was that such composite pictures might perhaps support the remarkable assertions being made at that time by Cesare Lombroso, the Italian psychiatrist and criminologist. In his book *L'uomo Delinquente* Lombroso had suggested that 'the criminal population' had a higher percentage of physical, nervous and mental anomalies than non-criminals. Criminals showed in their faces as well as their bodies what Lombroso liked to call the 'stigmata of degeneracy', due partly, he said, to degenerative and partly to atavistic characteristics. The criminal, to him, was a special type, 'lying midway between the lunatic and the savage'. If, as Lombroso believed, criminal tendencies were constitutional, then, Galton argued, they might be removed from the population by selective breeding. Galton's composite pictures of the 'criminal type' proved, in fact, to be no more convincing than his composite pictures of particular disease 'types'. Modern criminologists do not now believe that criminals belong to any single physical or psychological 'type', nor do they believe that there is any such thing as a 'constitutionally criminal type'. Many researchers, on the other hand, have been impressed by the strikingly similar characteristics of the psychological and emotional *backgrounds* of many criminals, and have generally concluded that criminals are not born but made.

On the question of professional faces, however, all we can do at the present is to confound or support our personal prejudices by considering as many cases as possible from different occupational groups, ask ourselves if we can discover any common elements, and, if so, reflect on their possible causes. Perhaps we can draw our own conclusions from the collection of portraits which follow.

Clearly, a comparison of this limited kind cannot be considered in any sense a scientific test of the hypothesis of 'professional similarity', but the reader may find the exercise an interesting one, and it may suggest to him an alternative and more convincing way of investigating this whole important area of research.

Our discussion so far has, by implication, been concerned only with static portraits and has neglected entirely to consider the transient, fleeting movements which occur in real faces. It is just such movements which are, as the old physiognomists often failed to realise, so crucial to the individual character of a face. It may very well be that the real distinguishing quality of the Field-Marshal's face is not so much its architecture, as displayed by a portrait, as its tension or relaxation, its movement or its lack of movement —qualities which could be assessed only in a direct confrontation in real life, or perhaps in a moving-film or television record. As we shall see in the next chapter, for successful judgement we need a great deal more than a simple snapshot portrait. Perhaps, therefore, the problem for future research should be to look for characteristic professional gestures, movements, and fleeting expressions and not for 'professional anatomy'.

The reader is invited to try to judge the professions, the identities and perhaps the nationalities of the men whose portraits follow in random order, over the next few pages. All of them have achieved distinction in their own profession—and some of them (as so often happens with genius) have made their mark in more than one field of activity. A key, identifying their professions, their names and their nationalities will be found on pages 255–257.

The following groups are represented:
Writers and poets
Artists
Composers
Philanthropists
Financiers
Monarchs
Politicians
Generals
Explorers
Scientists and philosophers
Social reformers

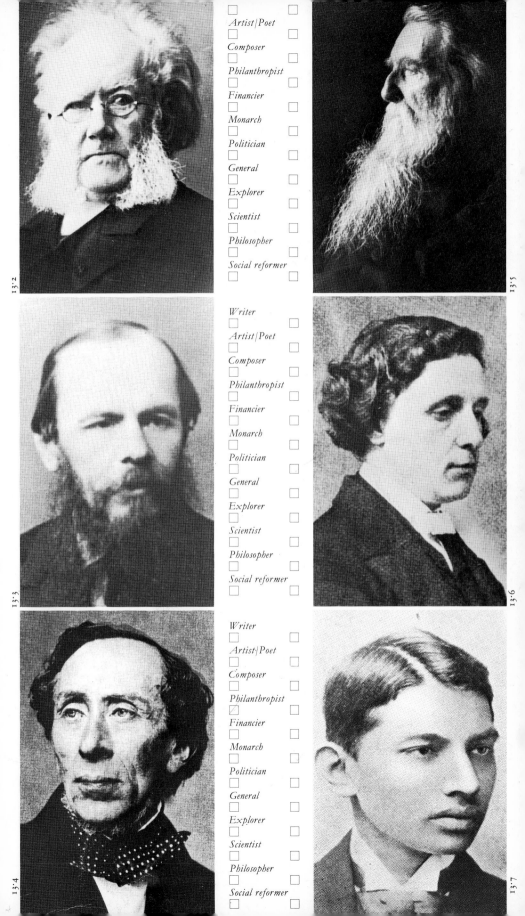

13·2

Artist/Poet ☐ ☐
Composer ☐ ☐
Philanthropist ☐ ☐
Financier ☐ ☐
Monarch ☐ ☐
Politician ☐ ☐
General ☐ ☐
Explorer ☐ ☐
Scientist ☐ ☐
Philosopher ☐ ☐
Social reformer ☐ ☐

13·5

13·3

Writer ☐ ☐
Artist/Poet ☐ ☐
Composer ☐ ☐
Philanthropist ☐ ☐
Financier ☐ ☐
Monarch ☐ ☐
Politician ☐ ☐
General ☐ ☐
Explorer ☐ ☐
Scientist ☐ ☐
Philosopher ☐ ☐
Social reformer ☐ ☐

13·6

13·4

Writer ☐ ☐
Artist/Poet ☐ ☐
Composer ☐ ☐
Philanthropist ☑ ☐
Financier ☐ ☐
Monarch ☐ ☐
Politician ☐ ☐
General ☐ ☐
Explorer ☐ ☐
Scientist ☐ ☐
Philosopher ☐ ☐
Social reformer ☐ ☐

13·7

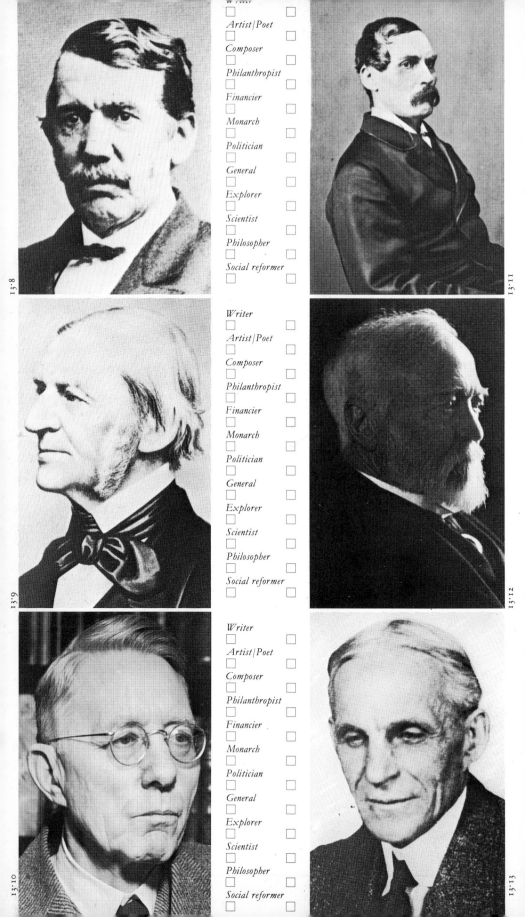

13·8

13·9

13·10

13·11

13·12

13·13

Writer ☐ ☐
Artist/Poet ☐ ☐
Composer ☐ ☐
Philanthropist ☐ ☐
Financier ☐ ☐
Monarch ☐ ☐
Politician ☐ ☐
General ☐ ☐
Explorer ☐ ☐
Scientist ☐ ☐
Philosopher ☐ ☐
Social reformer ☐ ☐

Writer ☐ ☐
Artist/Poet ☐ ☐
Composer ☐ ☐
Philanthropist ☐ ☐
Financier ☐ ☐
Monarch ☐ ☐
Politician ☐ ☐
General ☐ ☐
Explorer ☐ ☐
Scientist ☐ ☐
Philosopher ☐ ☐
Social reformer ☐ ☐

Writer ☐ ☐
Artist/Poet ☐ ☐
Composer ☐ ☐
Philanthropist ☐ ☐
Financier ☐ ☐
Monarch ☐ ☐
Politician ☐ ☐
General ☐ ☐
Explorer ☐ ☐
Scientist ☐ ☐
Philosopher ☐ ☐
Social reformer ☐ ☐

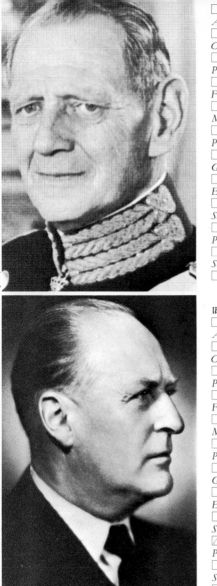

13·14

13·15

13·16

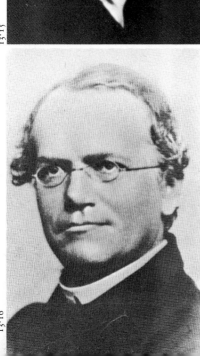

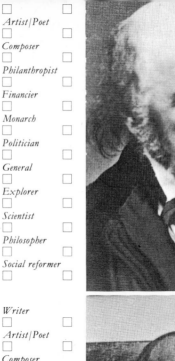

13·17

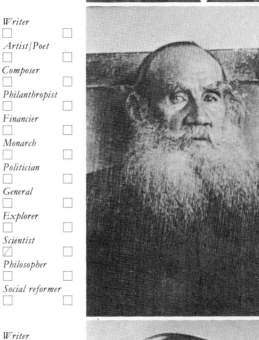

13·18

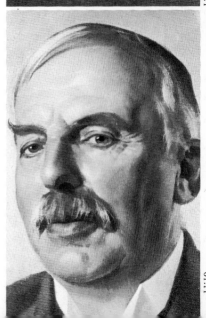

13·19

	□	Artist/Poet	□
	□	Composer	□
	□	Philanthropist	□
	□	Financier	□
	□	Monarch	□
	□	Politician	□
	□	General	□
	□	Explorer	□
	□	Scientist	□
	□	Philosopher	□
	□	Social reformer	□

	□	Writer	
	□	Artist/Poet	□
	□	Composer	□
	□	Philanthropist	□
	□	Financier	□
	□	Monarch	□
	□	Politician	□
	□	General	□
	□	Explorer	□
	☑	Scientist	□
	□	Philosopher	
	□	Social reformer	

	□	Writer	
	□	Artist/Poet	□
	□	Composer	□
	□	Philanthropist	□
	□	Financier	□
	□	Monarch	□
	□	Politician	□
	□	General	□
	□	Explorer	□
	□	Scientist	□
	□	Philosopher	□
	□	Social reformer	

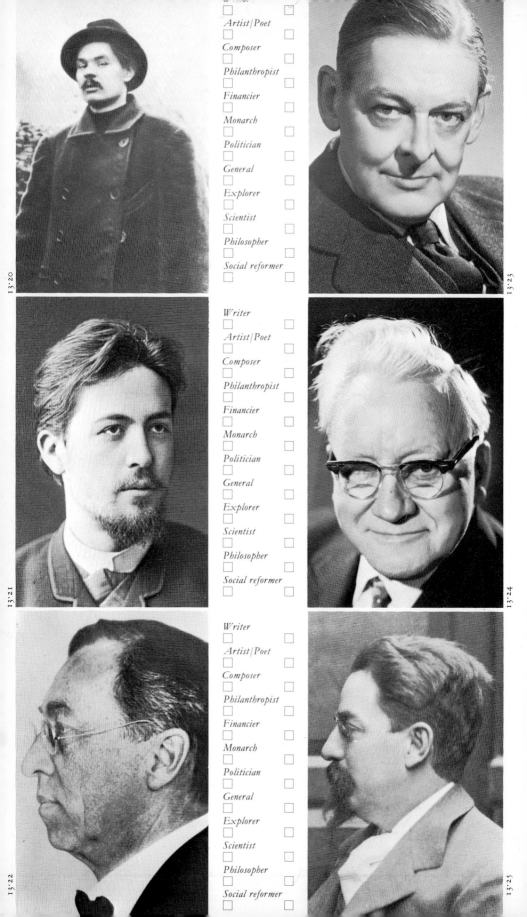

13·20

13·21

13·22

13·23

13·24

13·25

Artist/Poet
Composer
Philanthropist
Financier
Monarch
Politician
General
Explorer
Scientist
Philosopher
Social reformer

Writer
Artist/Poet
Composer
Philanthropist
Financier
Monarch
Politician
General
Explorer
Scientist
Philosopher
Social reformer

Writer
Artist/Poet
Composer
Philanthropist
Financier
Monarch
Politician
General
Explorer
Scientist
Philosopher
Social reformer

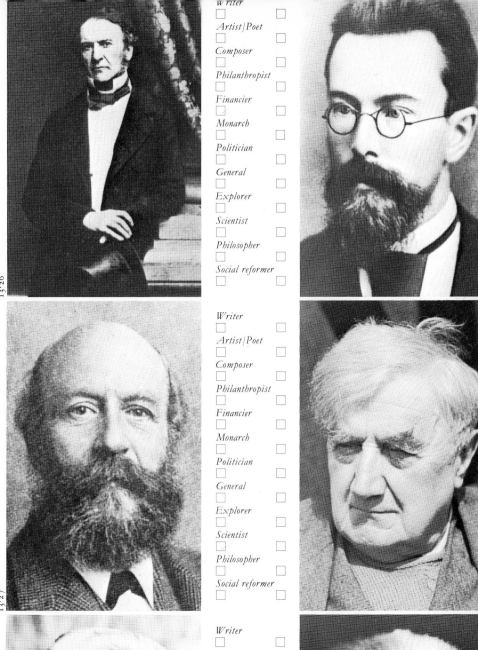

13·26

13·27

13·28

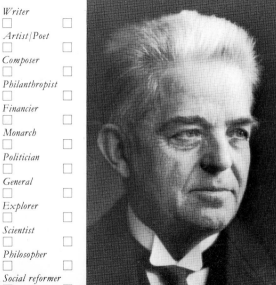

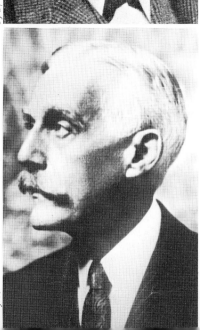

13·29

13·30

13·31

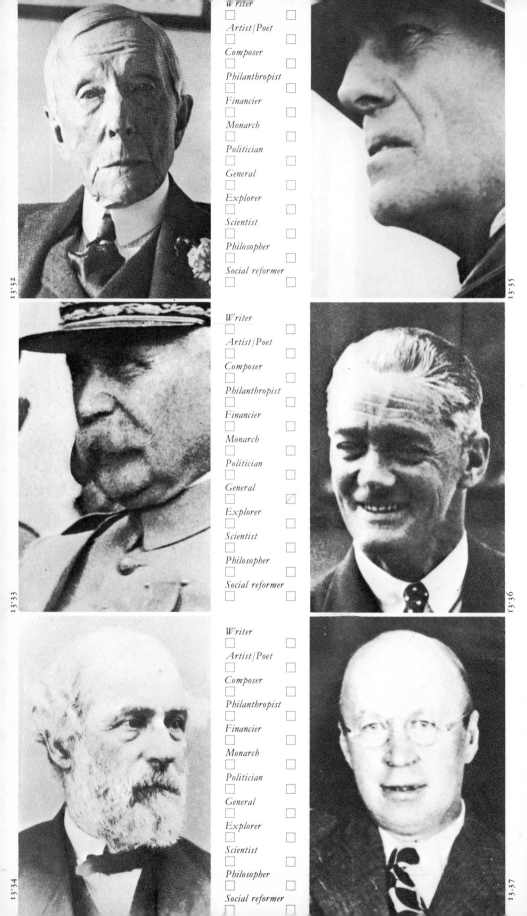

13·32

13·35

13·33

13·36

13·34

13·37

Writer ☐ ☐
Artist/Poet ☐ ☐
Composer ☐ ☐
Philanthropist ☐ ☐
Financier ☐ ☐
Monarch ☐ ☐
Politician ☐ ☐
General ☐ ☐
Explorer ☐ ☐
Scientist ☐ ☐
Philosopher ☐ ☐
Social reformer ☐ ☐

Writer ☐ ☐
Artist/Poet ☐ ☐
Composer ☐ ☐
Philanthropist ☐ ☐
Financier ☐ ☐
Monarch ☐ ☐
Politician ☐ ☐
General ☐ ☑
Explorer ☐ ☐
Scientist ☐ ☐
Philosopher ☐ ☐
Social reformer ☐ ☐

Writer ☐ ☐
Artist/Poet ☐ ☐
Composer ☐ ☐
Philanthropist ☐ ☐
Financier ☐ ☐
Monarch ☐ ☐
Politician ☐ ☐
General ☐ ☐
Explorer ☐ ☐
Scientist ☐ ☐
Philosopher ☐ ☐
Social reformer ☐ ☐

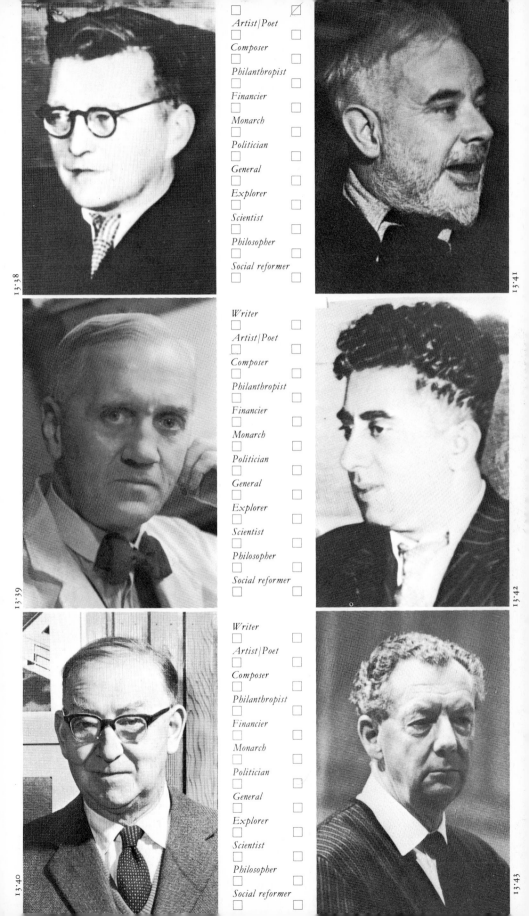

13·38

13·39

13·40

13·41

13·42

13·43

Artist/Poet ☑
Composer
Philanthropist
Financier
Monarch
Politician
General
Explorer
Scientist
Philosopher
Social reformer

Writer
Artist/Poet
Composer
Philanthropist
Financier
Monarch
Politician
General
Explorer
Scientist
Philosopher
Social reformer

Writer
Artist/Poet
Composer
Philanthropist
Financier
Monarch
Politician
General
Explorer
Scientist
Philosopher
Social reformer

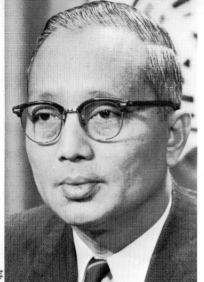

Artist/Poet

Composer

Philanthropist

Financier

Monarch

Politician

General

Explorer

Scientist

Philosopher

Social reformer

13·02 Writer
Henrik Ibsen 1828–1906
Norwegian dramatist, poet,
outstanding pioneer of social
drama
13·03 Writer
F. M. Dostoyevsky
1821–1881
Russian novelist, journalist,
outstanding writer of realist
fiction
13·04 Writer
Hans Andersen 1805–1875
Danish writer of fairy-tales
13·05 Writer
John Ruskin 1819–1900
English author and art-critic.
Writer on beauty and champion
of pre-Raphaelites
13·06 Writer
Charles Dodgson 1832–1898
'Lewis Carroll' : English writer
of children's books, notably
Alice in Wonderland
13·07 Politician
Mohandas Gandhi
1869–1948
Indian leader and patriot,
lawyer, moral teacher, social
reformer
13·08 Explorer
David Livingstone
1813–1873
Scottish missionary and
traveller

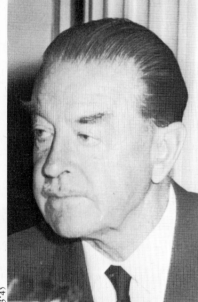

Writer

Artist/Poet

Composer

Philanthropist

Financier

Monarch

Politician

General

Explorer

Scientist

Philosopher

Social reformer

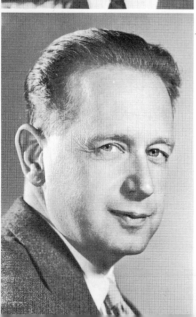

Writer

Artist/Poet

Composer

Philanthropist

Financier

Monarch

Politician

General

Explorer

Scientist

Philosopher

Social reformer

13·09 Writer
Ralph Waldo Emerson
1803–1882
American poet and essayist.
Great friend of Carlyle. Made
plea for individual consciousness
as supreme judge in spiritual
matters

13·10 Writer
Johannes Jensen 1873–1950
Danish novelist, essayist, poet,
traveller, Nobel prizewinner

13·11 Explorer
Sir R. F. Burton 1829–1890
English explorer, Consul,
translator of Arabian Nights

13·12 Financier/
Philanthropist
Andrew Carnegie 1835–1919
Scottish ironmaster and
philanthropist. Benefactions
exceeded £70 million

13·13 Financier
Henry Ford 1863–1947
American motor manufacturer.
Pioneered the 'assembly-line'.
Tried to negotiate European
peace 1915

13·14 Monarch
King Frederik of Denmark
1899–1972

13·15 Monarch
King Olav of Norway
b. 1903

13·16 Scientist
Gregor Mendel 1822–1884
Austrian biologist; pioneer of
genetics

13·17 Writer
Edward Fitzgerald
1809–1883
English scholar and poet.
Translator of Rubaiyat of Omar
Khayyam

13·18 Writer
Leo Tolstoi 1828–1910
Russian Count. Writer,
aesthetic philosopher, moralist
and mystic. Great novelist.
Author of War and Peace

13·19 Scientist
Ernest Rutherford
1871–1937
English scientist. Pioneer of
radioactivity and first to
recognise nuclear nature of the
atom

13·20 Writer
Maxim Gorki 1868–1936
Russian novelist and revolu-
tionary. Sponsored 'social
realism' as an official art form

13·21 Writer
Anton Chekhov 1860–1904
Russian playwright, author and
qualified physician. Inspired
whole school of writers

13·22 Artist
Vasily Kandinsky 1866–1944
Russian painter. Founded
Russian Academy. Abstract
theories exerted great influence
on European art

13·23 Writer
T. S. Eliot 1888–1965
American born British poet,
critic and dramatist. Author of
The Waste Land *and* Murder
in the Cathedral

13·24 Politician
Herbert Morrison
1888–1965
British politician. Formidable social legislator and reformer and leader of House of Commons
13·25 Social reformer
Sidney Webb 1859–1947
English social reformer; social historian and economist
13·26 Politician
William Gladstone
1809–1898
British liberal statesman; long record of successful, practical legislation
13·27 Financier/ Philanthropist
George Cadbury 1839–1922
English Quaker industrialist, newspaper proprietor and social reformer. Founded model village of Bournville
13·28 Politician
Andrew William Mellon
1855–1937
American politician, one of richest men in America. Made controversial fiscal reform. Ambassador to UK
13·29 Composer
N. A. Rimsky-Korsakov
1844–1908
Russian composer; teacher of Stravinsky

13·30 Composer
Ralph Vaughan-Williams
1872–1958
English composer; leader of English folksong movement. Operas notable for concern with moral issues of contemporary life
13·31 Composer
Carl Nielsen 1865–1931
Danish composer
13·32 Financier/ Philanthropist
J. D. Rockefeller 1839–1937
American millionaire oil monopolist and philanthropist. Gave away over 500 million dollars 'to promote the well-being of mankind'
13·33 General
Marshal Pétain 1856–1951
French soldier. Sentenced to death for treason as collaborationist
13·34 General
Robert E. Lee 1807–1870
American General. Masterly strategist of Confederate forces in Civil War
13·35 General
George Patton 1885–1945
American General: led brilliant campaign through France at head of Third Army
13·36 Financier
William Richard Morris
(Lord Nuffield) 1877–1963
English motor manufacturer and financier

13·37 Composer
S. Prokofiev 1891–1955
Russian composer and pianist.
Began to compose music at age of
five and first opera at age of nine
13·38 Composer
S. Shostakovich b. 1906
Russian composer. Experimental
style, officially criticised
13·39 Scientist
Sir Alexander Fleming
1881–1955
Scottish bacteriologist and
discoverer of penicillin; 1945
Nobel prizewinner for medicine
13·40 Scientist
Sir John Cockcroft
1897–1967
English physicist; won Nobel
Prize for physics in 1951
13·41 Philosopher
C. E. M. Joad 1891–1953
English philosopher and writer.
Did much to popularise
philosophy
13·42 Composer
Aram Ilyich Khachaturyan
b. 1903
Russian composer

13·43 Composer
Benjamin Britten b. 1913
English composer, especially of
opera, and occasional conductor
13·44 Politician
U Thant b. 1909
Burmese politician; Secretary-
General of the United Nations
13·45 General
Field-Marshal The Earl
Alexander 1891–1969
British General. C. in C.
Allied Armies in Italy
1944–45
13·46 Politician
Dag Hammarskjold
1905–1961
Swedish politician; Secretary-
General of the United Nations

14 The art of judgement

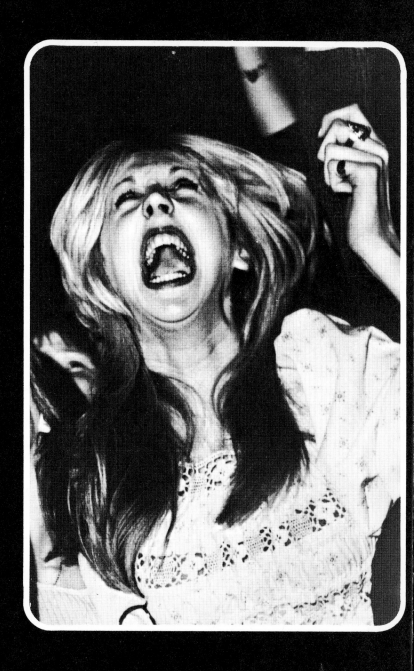

'There's no art to find the mind's construction in the face.'
Or so it seemed to Shakespeare's Duncan. Yet few of us
would agree with him. We know that we can assess people
adequately, that we can judge their feelings, sense their
cupidity, weigh their abilities and their weaknesses. We
rarely find difficulty, for example, in recognising the anger
or the happiness or the despair in a man's face. We know we
are right, and often, quite probably, we are. *Emotions* and
feelings we can certainly judge, whatever Shakespeare may
have said, for the very good reason that the basic mechanisms of emotional expression, as well as the means to recognise them, are, to a high degree, innate in our nature; there
is little need for us to learn, during our lifetime, how to
express them or how to recognise them. Some of the most
striking evidence that this is the case has come from studies
of children born blind; they can laugh and cry in a perfectly
ordinary way, without any opportunity for imitation from
the sight of family and friends. It is true, however, that the
subtlety of their expression does not continue to extend and
develop much after the age of four or five, as it does in the
majority of children. Most children go on to extend their
powers of expression very rapidly indeed, and soon display
astonishing ability to make their meaning clear. A six-year-
old, for example, can express defiance and suspicion in quite
distinct ways. Children's ability to recognise emotion, too,
develops rapidly and surprisingly early; Buhler and Hetzer
found that even five-month-old babies could distinguish
easily between an angry and a smiling face.

Not only are the basic mechanisms of emotion innate,
they also seem to be quite universal. As Darwin discovered,
most emotions have standard forms of expression which are
common to all members of the species. The whole of mankind is instantly sensitive to the smile: its meaning is universally recognised and understood. Crying in pain, weeping
in sorrow, scowling in anger—all of these take much the
same form throughout the world. Even more subtle feelings
like boredom and puzzlement seem to take remarkably
similar facial forms everywhere. There seem to be no boun-
daries of race or nationality in the field of emotional recognition. The Greeks are just as successful as Americans at
recognising the emotions in American faces. And so are the

Opposite:
*Many emotions are easy
enough to recognise, but
only if we know the
situation in which they
arise*

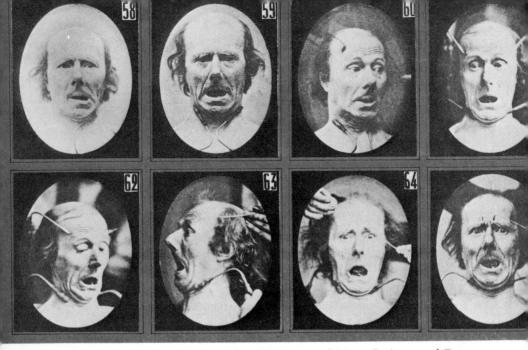

people of Brazil and Japan and New Guinea and Borneo—as recent research has made quite clear.

The study of the nature of the basic mechanisms of emotion has been undertaken in many different—and sometimes very curious—ways. The nineteenth-century physiologist Duchenne, for example, collected heads from the guillotine in Paris and applied electric currents to their facial nerves. It did not take him long to discover that this was not a very satisfactory form of experimentation since the muscles and nerves stayed active for only two or three hours after death. He continued his electrical experiments with the cooperation of an old almshouse patient who could not feel pain in his face. Duchenne's conclusion from these experiments—that single expressions such as the smile are caused by the action of single facial nerves—has not been supported by later research, which has demonstrated the extreme subtlety and complexity of the nervous control of expressions—a subtlety described in 1806 by Sir Charles Bell, the great Edinburgh anatomist, as 'the most remarkable in the whole extent of nature.' His classic work, *The Anatomy and Philosophy of Expression*, in which he illustrated with his own beautiful drawings the forms and mechanisms of the major expressions, remained a standard text for artists until comparatively recent times. As Bell explained,

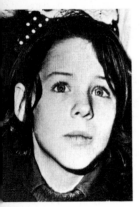

it is because many of our emotional expressions are brought about by entirely automatic bodily processes that we usually find it impossible to conceal them. The sudden blush of shame, like the pallor of fear, is produced by the 'autonomic' sector of the nervous system, which is completely beyond our control. It is now known that when a sudden emergency arises, adrenalin is released into the blood and the small blood vessels immediately contract, losing their blood and causing the face to grow pale. At the same time the heart beats faster, the throat becomes tense—to keep the breathing passages open during the expected crisis—and the corners of the mouth are pulled back quite automatically for the same purpose. All of these changes coalesce to produce 'the face of fear'—an expression which is instinctively recognised by all who see it.

Because the actual physical processes of the more subtle emotions have proved so complex and difficult to disentangle, some researchers went on to use an entirely different technique of analysis. The psychologist Piderit showed people portrait drawings of many different emotional states, and asked them to name the emotions they could see. By careful modifications of these drawings he was soon able to discover the muscular and facial positions which were crucial for the recognition of a particular emotion. In more recent times photographs of actors simulating emotions of various kinds have been used. One rather unexpected discovery from this recent work has been that people can judge *simulated* emotions much more readily than they can genuine emotions: the emotional conventions of expression of the stage and screen are evidently larger-than-life and much more stereotyped than the genuine, uncontrived expressions of ordinary life.

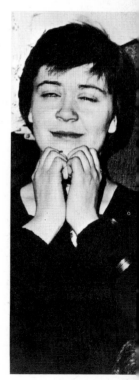

Unfortunately, most of these early experiments were undertaken with static portraits of one kind or another and, as we shall see, it is movement which is the essence of expression. Some of our best guides to a person's feelings—as indeed to intentions—come from the movements he makes. In his research in America, Birdwhistell has recently discovered several particularly significant movements which a careful observer can sometimes detect. Couples in love, for example, tend to cock their heads about and make

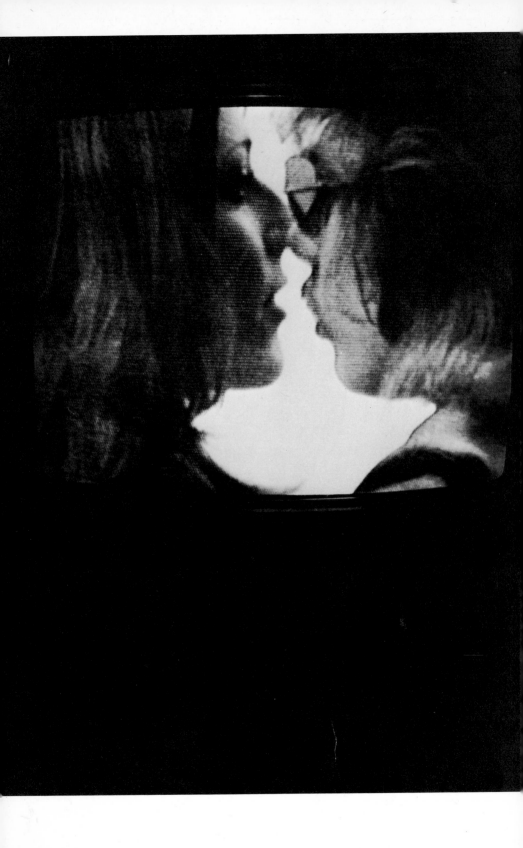

small, peculiar facial movements as they gaze into each other's eyes; their facial muscles become more taut, their skin flushed or pale, their eyes clearer and brighter. Furthermore, if we are prepared to look closely enough we will see changes and movements *within* the eyes themselves—a fact that was recognised at least a thousand years ago, in a rather different context, by the jade-dealers of the Orient, who veiled their eyes during bargaining so that the dilation of their pupils would not betray their excitement over a particularly fine piece of jewellery. Some of them even wore crude dark spectacles in order to mask this quite involuntary sign of enthusiasm, and so, it was hoped, avoid any increase in the trader's asking price. Not only does the pupil dilate, however, when we look at something pleasant, it promptly reduces again when we turn our eye to something less agreeable, or even when an unpleasant thought enters our mind. The American psychologist Eckhard Hess has constructed a 'pupillometer' for measuring these changes in our eyes when we get excited. It is a much more sensitive and effective method, he believes, than the 'lie-detector' as an indicator of our emotional state. The lie-detector simply registers the *presence* of emotional excitement; it does not reveal the nature of the emotion.

But the way we move the whole eye may be very revealing too. Recent research has shown that careful study of eye movements and direction of gaze can tell us a great deal. As Argyle has discovered, we are all highly skilled in using our eye movements to show our partner that we are angry, bored or happy, or that we are attracted by him, or even that we have a strong urge to dominate him. Our eye movements also operate in a more subtle way to regulate and maintain the stability and continuity of our interaction with another person. When, for example, X is talking, he may tend not to look directly into Y's eyes. Only when he is coming to the end of what he has to say does he look at Y again and so, unwittingly, give the signal that he is finishing and that the time has come for Y to begin talking. Eye-movements of this kind, too, play an important part in controlling the level of intimacy which two people allow to develop between themselves. If at any particular moment intimacy seems to be getting too great, then eye-contact is

Opposite.
Birdwhistell has found that couples in love make small but peculiar movements of their heads and faces as they gaze into each other's eyes

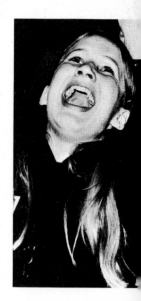

voluntarily renounced by the couple and they look away from each other. If more intimacy seems mutually welcome, then more gazing into each other's eyes—and often, between lovers, even from eye to eye—will be permitted. For most ordinary contacts and conversations, however, there seems to be an acceptable 'equilibrium level' of intimacy which is controlled by this kind of 'eye-contact' as well as by several other factors, such as physical closeness to the other person, the intimacy of the topic of conversation itself, and even tone of voice. When any single one of these factors is altered—for example by two people in conversation being pushed closer together in an elevator—then there will be a compensatory change to restore the old acceptable level of equilibrium: the eyes of both parties will be suddenly averted and conversation suddenly stopped. By contrast, couples who are forced further apart manage to keep up their intimacy by longer periods of mutual eye-gazing. Sex seems to influence the way the eyes are used. When women talk they gaze into the eyes of their companions; men, on the other hand, are much more likely to 'address the air' around the other person. This may explain why women are so often more accurate in their judgements of people: they have more opportunity to assess the effect of their words while they are in conversation. And as T. H. Pear has explained, the people who are most successful in judging the feelings and characters of others are often those who 'prod' the other person with words and then carefully watch their effect. There are probably other reasons, of course, for women's superior judgement; perhaps their more vulnerable social position, in the past at least, has made them more sensitive to, and more conscious of, signs of *genuine* feeling and affection.

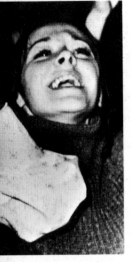

Another point has emerged from recent research on emotional recognition—and this is the crucial part played by physical context and surroundings in the conclusions we reach about a person's feelings—and even about his or her personality. One notable study showed that people are judged more attractive when they are seen in rooms which are themselves aesthetically pleasing. It is easy to imagine how much more influential would be the more intimate framework provided by hair and dress and ornament. Even

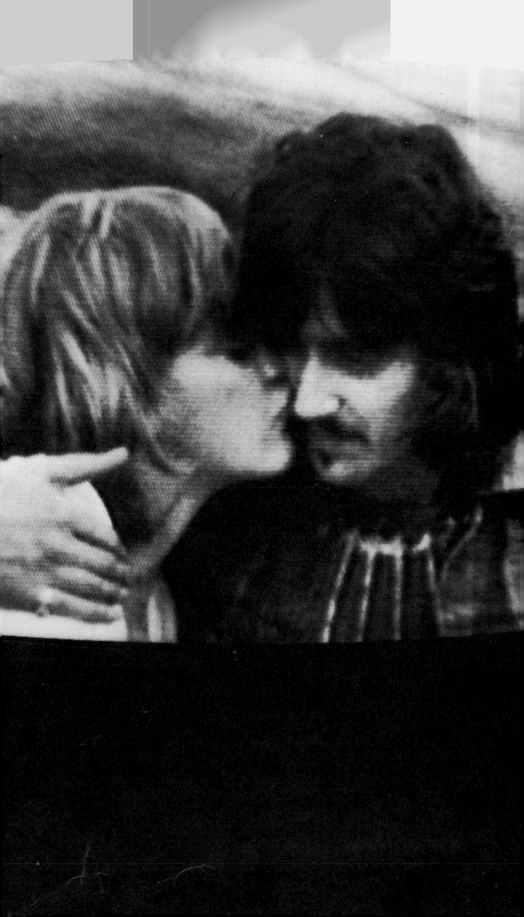

the correct recognition of emotion depends on knowing the physical context. The photograph illustrates this point. It is difficult to put a name to the emotion on the faces of the teenagers in the isolated pictures—it might equally well be horror, shock or even pain. When we see, however, that this face is one of a group of teenagers at a Beatles concert the true emotion of ecstatic bliss is easy to recognise. The whole task of recognition in this case is, of course, made doubly difficult because the image is not in natural motion, as it would certainly be in ordinary everyday experience. It is interesting to see how facial expression takes on quite different meanings in different surroundings. The interpretation of a smile depends a great deal on whether it is seen in a church or a pub, a sales interview or a court of law.

Not only do we require information about the physical background, however, we need contextual information of another and more subtle kind, about social class and background, for example. Does this person come from a stratum of society where too much free expression is frowned upon? Influences of this kind may be strong. Otto Klineberg tells how young Chinese girls used to be admonished, 'Do not show your unhappiness easily; don't smile easily; when you smile don't let your teeth be seen.' A perfectly happy Chinese girl might therefore easily be recognised as happy by her fellow villagers but seem shy, reserved, even unhappy, to a visiting European. In research in Britain, Sir Cyril Burt discovered wide social differences in acceptable standards of expressiveness—and Honkavaara found that even educational level was important:

> In educated families negative and violent emotions are usually inhibited, yet it seems that the children of these families recognise them better than those children of less intellectual parents who display their emotions freely.

This whole question of acceptable levels of expressiveness has been much neglected in discussions about emotion—and yet it is crucial to any consideration of accuracy of judgement. There is no doubt that some individuals, perhaps by training, perhaps by temperament, are what we can only describe as 'facialisers'—pouring their every emotion into their active, animated faces. Others, perhaps best described as 'internalisers', seem, either by constitution,

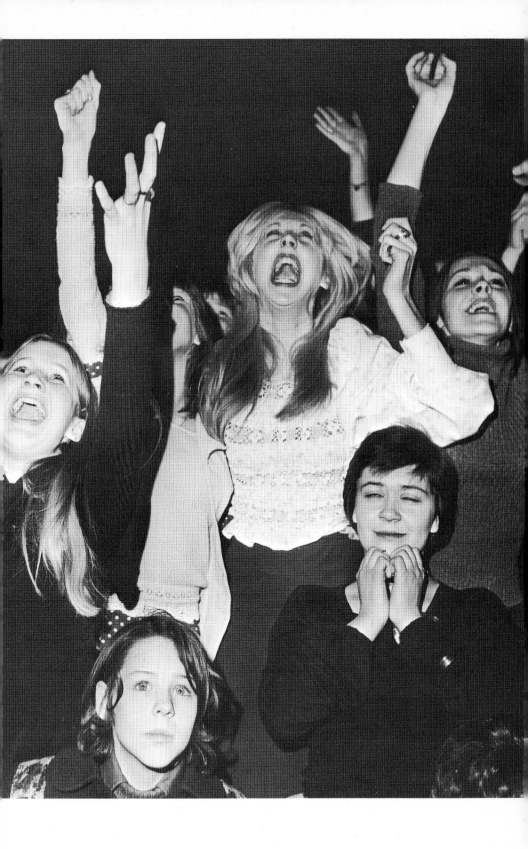

habit or preference—or perhaps simply by downright determination—able to suppress their outward facial show. It is clear that it is desirable to know whether we are dealing with a 'facialiser' or an 'internaliser' before we start drawing too many conclusions about a person's emotions. But there is a further environmental effect to be considered—and this is occupational context. Receptionists and air-hostesses, for example, are expected, as part of their jobs, to smile readily and convincingly to everyone, whatever their mood. How they really feel might be extremely difficult to assess.

There are still more environmental factors to consider when assessing the significance of facial expression. As Bird-whistell discovered, even *regional differences* in expressiveness need to be taken into account. He found differences in the readiness to smile in different parts of the United States. There are 'high smile areas', he discovered, in the Deep South. In Western New York State, by contrast, the smile is much less in evidence. And in the States bordering the Great Lakes a person smiling with an ease perfectly proper in the South might well find himself challenged to explain 'what he finds so funny'.

And yet, in spite of all these hazards and difficulties, we still succeed remarkably well in judging other people's feelings. Nature has equipped us well for social life. Our successful adaptation has been achieved only by the growth of considerable powers of intuition and a well-developed capacity for empathy—for fellow-feeling with our neigh-bours. We have acquired a remarkable sensitivity to the signals generated by other people—and of many of these we are not even consciously aware. Some of these are quite subtle signals arising from movement and gesture, from speech and behaviour, as well as from the face itself.

The same is undoubtedly true of our attempts at the assessment of the more durable aspects of human nature—qualities of character, temperament and personality. Great accuracy is possible. But here we need more time. Signifi-cant qualities of character are not in the least likely to be perceived in a brief momentary glance. Time is needed to observe the whole sequence of behaviour—the movements, the gestures, the fidgets—above all else, the words spoken. All of these must be carefully weighed and assessed in

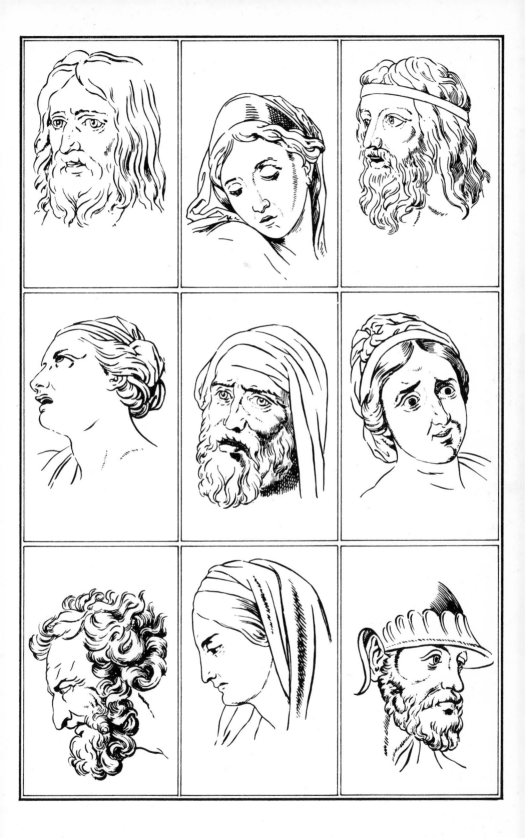

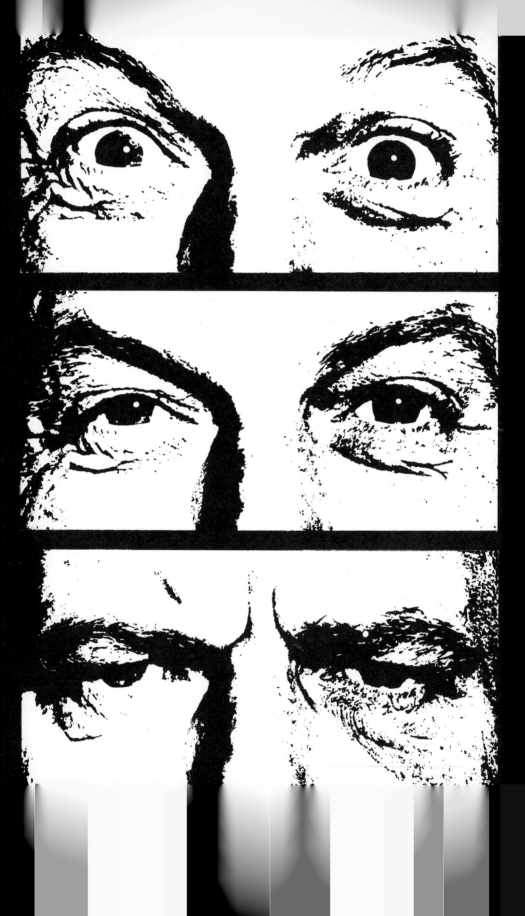

relation to the particular context, physical and social, in which we encounter them.

If we are tempted to judge from a snapshot or from a moment's brief glimpse of a face—and the temptation is sometimes a strong one—then we shall certainly be over-impressed by unimportant and trivial detail. Research by Thornton has shown, for example, that faces with spectacles might well be judged five per cent more intelligent than the same faces seen without spectacles. A similarly erroneous boost seems to be provided by a smile. Research has also shown that we are highly susceptible to quite trivial changes in the small detail of a face. Slight differences in the spacing of facial features materially affect judgements of certain moral qualities. For example, a slight increase in the distance between the eyes causes a person to be judged more honest and reliable. Especially important seems to be the distance of the brows from the eyes: too close and they create a falsely 'malevolent' impression, too high, and they suggest open-mindedness and accessibility. And remarkably small changes in eyebrow height profoundly affect our conclusions about intelligence. Thickness of the brows, too, can be misleadingly impressive: heavy bushy brows often lead to a judgement of 'firmness and gravity'. The angle of the brows, again, seems much too influential. The person with steeply slanting brows which are high in the middle is all too often seen as 'menacing'—however gentle and benign his true personality. The shape of the mouth can easily lead to false conclusions, a narrow slit often creating a misleading impression of 'introversion'. Downward-drooping corners or even a droopy moustache, may easily lead to a quite false attribution of maliciousness.

Sometimes a small detail of a person's appearance can prompt us to endow him with a 'halo'. Something about his face, his manner, or his speech instantly pleases us. And all the research shows that every subsequent judgement we make about him will be excessively coloured by this favourable first impression. Each decision we make about his abilities, his social skills, his personality or his leadership will be much more favourable than it should have been. The converse also occurs: a poor first impression may unjusti-fiably depress all our subsequent judgements of a man's

Opposite:
*The positions and
movements of eyes and
eyebrows play a crucial
part in our decisions
about emotion and even
about personality*

merits. Another curious error sometimes arises by 'parataxis'. What occurs here is that the person we are judging happens to remind us of a person of similar appearance whom we have known in the past—someone perhaps who was highly significant in our life and about whom we felt strongly—a parent perhaps, or a loved one, or even a hated headmaster. The feelings we experienced years ago come flooding back into the present and attach themselves to this person in front of us now. Sometimes it happens that the person we are reminded of is none other than ourselves. So arises one of the most curious errors of all—the 'narcissistic error'. Anyone who shares our likes, our dislikes, our values—or especially perhaps some real or imagined feature of our appearance—is inevitably attractive to us. In consequence, he will usually be overestimated. It is interesting to see how this effect operates in business, politics and public affairs. Company Chairmen, even Prime Ministers and Presidents, often tend to surround themselves with men who are, in some way, images of themselves—even the facial resemblances can sometimes be remarkable. The practical consequences may, of course, be entirely beneficial, since it is much easier to understand and, presumably, all the more effectively control, people whom we like and with whom we can easily identify. Many useful and effective working teams are undoubtedly composed in this way.

Paradoxically, it is our overweening desire for rationality and logic which so often leads us into erroneous judgements about people. We seem to put ourselves under strong pressure to justify our decisions—if only to ourselves—to find reasons (or perhaps they are rationalisations) for our decisions. Perhaps this is why the idea of 'typing' people into neat, separate and distinct categories is so tempting. It is pleasant and reassuring to get people safely and neatly packaged and pigeon-holed. We know then how to behave with them, what to do, what postures to adopt. All sorts of categories come to mind—'foreigners', 'politicians', 'policemen', 'the upperclasses', 'old people', 'young people'. We each have our own private collection of stereotypes which perhaps we feel helps us to deal speedily and effectively with those we meet. Once we have a person safely typed and pigeon-holed we know what to expect. If a person is an 'old person' he is bound to be rigid, conservative and slow; if he is a 'young person' he is bound to be flexible, liberal and quick-witted. The question we must consider, however, is whether groupings of this kind have any real justification. Are such groups even homogeneous? Are all old people the same? Are all politicians cast in the same mould? The answer surely is that there are enormous variations within all human groups. The individuals we often try to gather together under one single label are, in fact, quite unique. And any attempt to force people into a mere half dozen categories is not going to do justice to the facts. Unfortunately, such 'stereotyping' is all too tempting. And there are some categories, such as 'nationality' and 'class', which seem to have a particular fascination. Each nationality and each social class seems somehow to be expected to have its own special and 'characteristic' personality. The facts, of course, totally contradict such beliefs. Yet a famous research study by Katz and Braly showed how even the most sensitive and intelligent people can be trapped into this kind of error. More than sixty per cent of the Princeton students who took part in the research were prepared to declare that 'All Englishmen are sportsmanlike', 'All Americans are enterprising' and even that 'All Italians are passionate'. This kind of error is often compounded by the further, quite common, but erroneous, belief that there are *national* styles in faces—that there is, for instance, a 'typically English' face. A man with such a face must necessarily be English, and therefore sportsmanlike, or so the argument goes.

Proneness to this sort of error varies, of course, from person to person. Some people—Milton Rokeach describes them as 'closed-minded'—seem particularly susceptible; they have no room for too many categories, and certainly no room for subtle intermediate categories: a man is either good or bad. When faced with any kind of uncertainty or ambiguity—about the colour of a man's skin, for example—they must rapidly decide on one colour or the other. The curious thing—as recent research has shown—is that such a person will usually decide on the attribute he happens to be prejudiced against. If he happens to have anti-negro feelings he will describe a person of intermediate skin colour as 'negro', and will promptly assign to him the full range of

what he believes to be 'negro' temperamental characteristics. If, on the other hand, he is anti-white he will see
the indefinite skin colour as white—and will not be in the
least surprised to find all the usual white man's characteristics.

We are sometimes tempted into another kind of error—
the so-called 'logical error'. This arises when we infer that a
particular quality *must* be present in this person because we
have detected the presence of another quality which we
believe unfailingly to go with it. Many people believe, for
example, that ability and energy go together; that those who
are intelligent are also inevitably hardworking and energetic.
Yet this association is by no means common, as any school-
teacher will confirm. Another error, of a somewhat similar
kind, arises from 'metaphorical generalisation'—jumping to
the conclusion, for example, that men with rough eyebrow
hairs must necessarily also possess a rough, rugged temperament. Of course, no one has ever succeeded in demon-
strating any relationship whatsoever between the physical
processes underlying rough hair growth and the psychological processes underlying brusqueness of manner. Yet
physiognomists have been telling us for centuries that such
relationships do exist and can be relied on—and we have
begun to believe them. Popular novelette writers often use
their readers' susceptibility to this kind of false inference in
order to add colour and life to their characters; their books,
too, like those of the physiognomists, are full of men with
firm, strong jaws who invariably display exactly the same
firmness and strength in their characters.

Equivalences of this kind are tempting and attractive—
indeed many of the ideas of the physiognomists are intel-
lectually attractive in themselves. Human nature *is* interesting, and the things people say about it, the words
writers write about it, tend in themselves to be interesting.
But this should not blind us where there is oversimplifica-
tion or mutual inconsistency—and there is much of both
to be found in the writings of the physiognomists. Neither
should we allow ourselves to be captivated by the welcome
feeling of certainty which simple physiognomic rules so
often seem to supply.

There is no doubt that people vary a great deal in their

success in judging character and personality. Some seem to be able to grasp the essential character of a person very quickly indeed.

But why is it that they are so successful? According to Harvard psychologist G. W. Allport, the secret lies in the particular nature of their own personality. Good judges, according to Allport, have a 'passion for the subjective'. They are prepared to treat their hunches seriously. They are often people with high aesthetic sensitivity, and often, too, fairly complicated people themselves—always as mentally sophisticated, Allport believes, as the people they judge successfully. Very often, too, they are introverts. This is a surprising discovery; one might well have expected the active social life of the extrovert to have given him richer and wider experience of other people—a keener sense of human differences. This, evidently, is not the case; an impressive amount of research data clearly indicates that introverts tend to judge other people more accurately than extroverts. The American O.S.S. found during their wartime studies, for example, that the best selectors of likely collaborators in enemy territory generally tended to be introverts themselves. It was not the men who scored best on tests of social ability, or of extroversion, but quiet, introverted logicians who usually drew the right conclusions.

However, perhaps we should be cautious about speaking of 'good' or 'bad' judges, as though a man's judgements of others were likely to be always right or always wrong. Much depends upon *who* is being judged. Success may well be greater, for example, where the judge has a great deal in common with the person he is assessing; not only do we admire more, we also *understand* more the people who are like ourselves. Much depends, too, on the qualities we are trying to assess. There are some characteristics—such as aggressiveness—which are easy enough to see; others, like altruism, are not nearly so visible. And it is not only qualities but *people* who vary in 'visibility'. Some people—Estes calls them 'open types'—are easy enough to assess; their hearts are cheerfully displayed for all to see. Others—the 'closed-types'—play their cards very close to the chest; they pose very real problems for those who would assess them. Fortunately, there are just as many frank 'facialisers' in the world who cheerfully provide the careful observer with plenty of clues.

There can be little doubt that the face plays a crucial part in our everyday assessment of our fellows. Not only does it enable us to identify transient emotions—flashes of pleasure and rage, disappointment and hatred—it can also help us to make useful judgements about more durable and lasting qualities of personality and character, provided, of course, that we are cautious and mindful of the potential errors we have discussed. Even a static portrait may give us some impression of a man's social setting—his place in the world. Such things are visible, of course, not so much from the skin and bone and features as from the trappings around the face—the frame, the clothing, the elaborations. Fortunately, we are rarely obliged to base our judgements on anything so insubstantial as a snapshot portrait or a momentary glimpse of a passing face. Much more often we have the opportunity to survey the whole person, to look for all-important clues in gestures, expressions and eye movements—a sudden

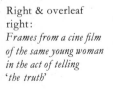

Right & overleaf right:
Frames from a cine film of the same young woman in the act of telling 'the truth'

and telling 'a lie'

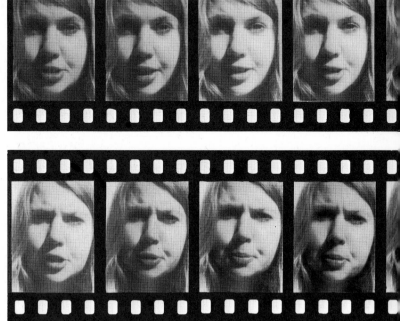

turning away, a pursing of the lips, a clenching of the teeth. And all of these movements acquire added significance when we have the opportunity to weigh them and assess them in relation to the context in which we see them, when we are able to know, for example, the restraining or facilitating effect of social background. Most important of all, of course, we usually have an opportunity to *talk* to the person about his likes and dislikes, his enthusiasms, his hopes and fears, his values, his ambitions. Again, we often have the opportunity to vary the context, to intervene, to discuss, challenge, or, as T. H. Pear suggests, to 'prod' the other person conversationally to see how he moves. In this way we can double and redouble the signals we receive, and we can begin to build up a collection of impressions from which a picture of personality can slowly emerge. The probability that this is a *true* picture will increase with every extra minute of time, with every extra word, every extra nod and fidget, every grimace and smile we are able to observe.

This kind of accuracy is achieved because much the most

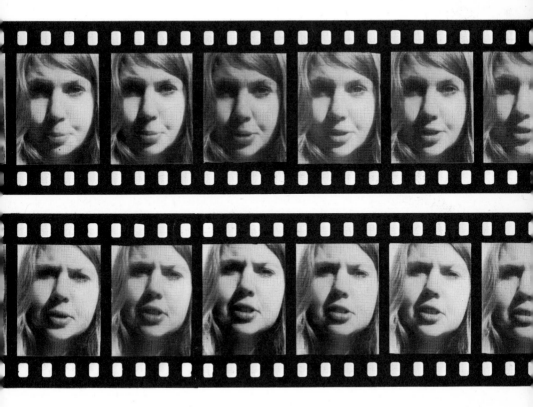

successful part of our judgement is *intuitive*; a lifetime of
social intercourse has left us sensitive and highly responsive
to quite subtle signals of which we are only barely conscious—or indeed of which we may be totally unaware.
Many of the most important of these signals arise from the
human face. But it is not the static sculpture of the face
which provides them. Nor is it the shapes, lines or colours
of its surface. It is the vital, active and above all the *moving*
face which tells us what we need to know.

It is certainly not the breadth of chin, the width of eye,
the length of nose which provide the all-important, vital
clues. Indeed, it would be better if we were to clear our
minds of lingering remembrances of old-fashioned rules
about weak chins and weak characters, high brows and high
intellects. It is natural enough—and reasonable enough—to
look, as men have looked for thousands of years, for simple,
straightforward rules of this kind, to provide us with
certainty in our judgements of character. But the certainty
we think we find in physiognomic rules, and the stereotypes

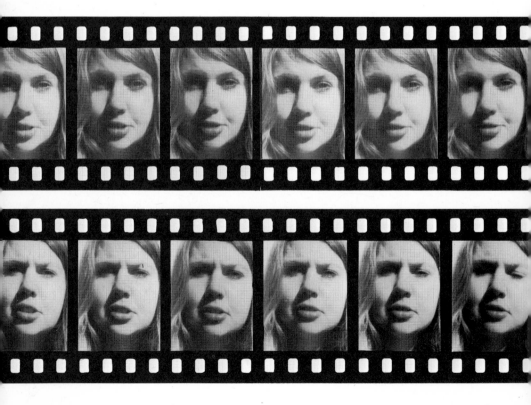

which spring from them, is false. It would be a pity if we
allowed ourselves to be misled by dogmatic rules and
sterile stereotypes which have never found the slightest
shred of scientific support. For to rely on these so-called
'rules' would be to nullify our undoubted natural intuitive
talents for appreciating, by the subtlest processes of empathy, the hearts and minds of our companions. The time is
not far distant, of course, when the equations linking face
and character will be written with certainty—when we shall
be able to relate truly accurate descriptions of facial forms,
textures and movements with genuinely objective measurements and analyses of personality. The science of personality
description is already well advanced: its achievements are
already impressive. We must await the development of an
entirely new technology of facial description and analysis
which matches in power and precision the science of
personality. Then we shall be able to pronounce with
certainty on the relationship of face and character. Then we
shall know whether, and to what degree, certain aspects of

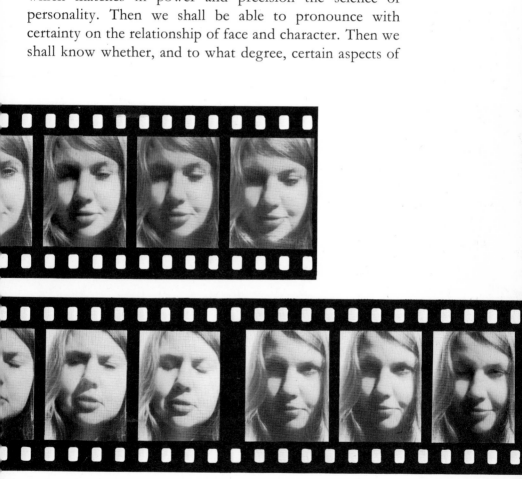

Right *'True' statement.
'He's a nice person',
while looking at a
portrait of Gandhi*

Right *'True' statement.
A different young
woman looking at the
same portrait of Gandhi*

Right and below
*'False' statement. The
same young women
saying 'He's a nice
person' while looking at
a portrait of Hitler*

*continued from previous
pages*

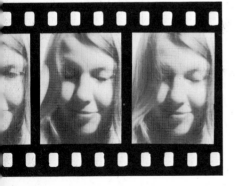

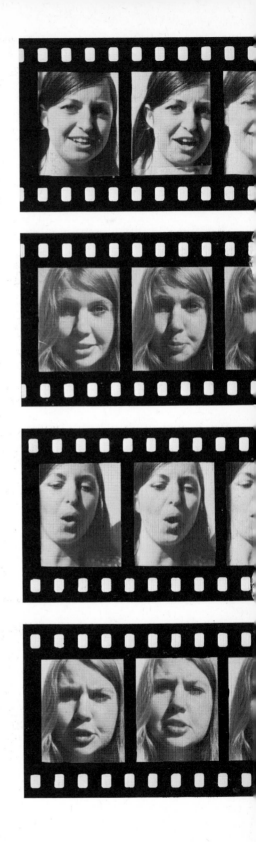

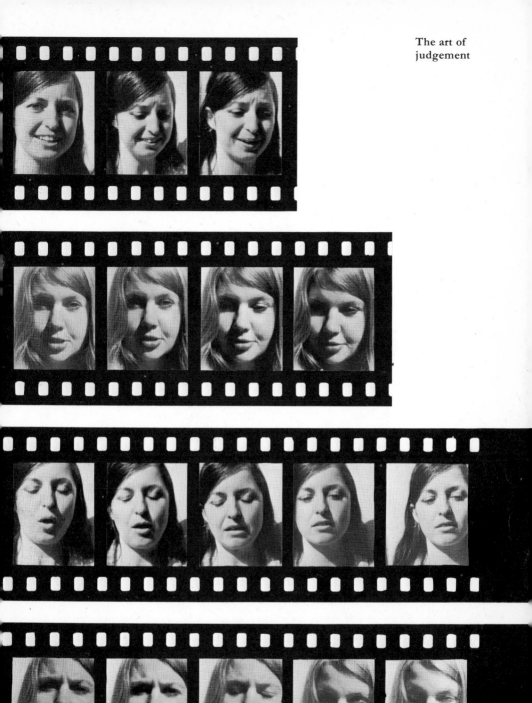

facial structure and movement are serviceable guides to personality and experience. Meanwhile, throughout our lives we shall continue to make our own personal judgements. And no harm could possibly follow our decisions if the act of making them were nothing more than a passive intellectual exercise—a pastime—like the judging of pictures at an exhibition. But the act of judging people is so very much more than this; it is an act of commitment to our fellow-men. So much of our behaviour towards people is crucially dependent on the way we see them, the way we instantaneously react to them.

It has been the message of this book that our impressions, our judgements and inevitably, therefore, our social behaviour are all too often determined by aspects of the human face which are trivial; that we are much too susceptible to the illusions, stereotypes and prejudices generated by these small details, and that the errors which spring from these effects are doubled and redoubled when we are confronted with the problem of judging faces out of their natural context. It is to the face, above all else, that we look for clues. It is in the face that we place our trust. The future—perhaps the very near future—will tell us whether our trust has been well-placed.

There are those who believe that man never has been, nor ever will be, completely knowable; that there is some divine mystery about human personality which it is at once improper and impossible to investigate. I reject this mystical view and insist that human personality and its external signs both can be and must be completely understood. The more explicitly the guiding principles of human experience and behaviour can be enunciated by future researchers, and the more effectively we can learn to apply these principles, the less will we be subject to the errors of facial misunderstanding which too often have blighted our personal, our industrial and even our international relationships. And the better we understand human personality and its outward signs, the freer we shall be to open ourselves to the possibility of friendship and love for our fellows. Such openness and mutual understanding are, without question, essential preconditions not only for our own emotional development and personal happiness but also, ultimately, for our survival as a unique, creative species.

Index

Acceptance of self 137
Acne treatment 128
Acromegaly (gigantism) 235, 237, 238, 239
Adolescents 23, 29, 128
Afghans 52, 115, 116–17
African tribes,
  art 174, 176, 178
  hair 37
  hats/head-dresses 108
  head elongation 46
  lip distortion 46, 49
  medicine men 166
  scarification 52, 53
  tattooing 54–5
Age, chronological/physiological 28–9
Ageing,
  premature 28
  processes 8, 23–6, 29, 31
  theories 26, 28–9
Alcohol excess, effect of 26, 234
Anaemia, facial indication of 237
Amazon tribes (Cobeus) 48
America see North America, South America, Indians, American
Ape skull 2, 4
Aristotle as physiognomist 181, 182, 192, 216, 217, 220
Artists,
  creating beauty standards 152, 153, 154
  face/torso parallel 174, 175–6, 178
  impressionists and beauty 156
  mathematical approach to beauty 140
Assyrians, ancient 54, 97
Asthenic physique 237, 243
Astrology 184–4, 186
Australian natives 43, 51
Avicenna, Arab physician 182, 218, 220

Baby,
  emotional expression 29, 259
  face of 4, 8, 24–5
  skull deformed for beauty 43–6
Balding 238
Beards,
  antipathy with wigs 100
  Biblical instructions 97
  British/Russian attempts to tax 98
  in North America 100, 103
  mourning sign 97
  red, sign of sin to Moslems 218
  sacredness of 98
  sign of profession 92
  touching significance of 98
  varieties and changing fashion 91, 92, 97–9, 100–3
  virility sign 97
Beauty,
  a highly personal experience 155
  ancient and modern ideals 142–3
  artists' approach to 140–1, 152–4, 156
  differing standards 43, 46, 155
  see also Lip deformation, Skull deformation etc
  factors influencing concept of 150–56
  film stars 156, 157
  male/female 146–9
  national differences 61–5
  philosophical concept of 142, 150, 155, 156
  proportions for 140–5
  psychological concepts of 142, 150–1
  score (Brislin's) 144, 145
  sexual aspects 150–1
  totality of experience 142, 150
Bedouin eyeball painting 48

Belladonna 21–2
Bell's palsy 236
Bhutan tribe preserving head of dead 162
Biblical references,
  to beards/hair 97, 98, 173
  to character in faces 181
  to classification of race 31
  to self torture and sacrifice 51
Birthmarks 126
Blushing 261
Bones, development of facial 4
  see also skull
Borneo tribes 51, 163
Brain
  bumps in phrenology 205–6
  functional areas 212
Brazil, lip distortion as beauty 46, 49
Britons, ancient, tattooing 54
Bunraku theatre 169
Burma theatrical mask 169
Burqua (veil) 116

Caste marking by tattoo 54
Caucasoid race 4, 31, 35
Ceruse 61, 63, 67, 68
Ceylon masks 116, 168, 169
Chadri (veil) 116
Character see Personality
Children,
  emotional expression 259
  resemblance to mother/father 201
  phrenologists' views on education 213
Chin,
  in Lavater's physiognomy 199, 220, 221
  surgery 132–3, 135
Chinese,
  culture 37–8, 169, 170, 266
  features 35, 37–8

Church, attitude to,
  cosmetic surgery 125
  fans 117
  hair 87
Cicatrisation 52, 53
Climate, effect on skin 25
Colour see Eye colour and Skin colour
Complexion, bad,
  concealed by patches 121–2
  treated by cosmetic surgery 128
Computer,
  correlation of features and character 229
  portrait of Abraham Lincoln 18–9
Congenital diseases corrected by cosmetic surgery 126–7
Convertible face 156
Corpse treatment 162–6
Cosmetic surgery,
  cost of 135
  early 125
  mediaeval 125
  modern use of 125–8, 130–2, 136–7
  personality regression following 136
Cosmetics,
  advertising 65, 72, 73, 74, 75–7
  ancient 60–5, 90–1
  cost of modern 75–6
  European changing fashions 65–73
  in classical poetry 61
  legal control of (Britain 1770) 69
  Ovid's advice 61
  male 48, 61, 63, 70, 73, 79, 87, 90
  Kama Sutra advice 65
  see also Wigs
  poisonous/harmful 68–9, 88
  purpose of,
    accentuating male/female features 21, 150–1
    bleaching skin colour 16
    indicated by adver-

tising appeals 75
nourishment and protec-
tion of skin 63, 73,
75, 76
ritual/magical 64–5,
67, 75
Suffering and sacrifice
75
Criminal faces 244,
282
Crows feet 25, 133
Crying 259
Cushing's syndrome
235, 236, 237

Death,
face at time of (facies
hippocratica) 181,
232, 233
funeral masks 166, 167
head retained after
162–6
wax mask cult of
Romans 182
Décolletage, exploita-
tion of 81
Della Porta, physiog-
nomist 186, 187,
192, 218, 220
Depression (melan-
cholia) face type 238
Diathesis 236
Disease see Illness
Drama masks 167–9

Ears,
and beauty 143, 144
145, 146
cosmetic surgery on
126, 127, 128
in love making 161
in physiognomy 217
piercing for beauty 48,
49
and race 38
East Indies, teeth
ritual 51
Egyptians, ancient,
beards and hair 81,
85, 87, 97
cosmetic use 63
funeral masks 166–7
power of eye 170
skull 35, 45, 46
tattooing 54
Elasticity of skin 8,
24–5

Elevativeness 223–4
Elizabethan cosmetics
and hair fashions
66–7, 85, 87, 100
Embryonic face 1
Emotion,
training to modify 266
of psychiatric cases
237–9
universality of expres-
sion 259–60
Emotional expression,
artists' impressions of
269
change in ageing 29, 31
differing social stan-
dards 266
experimental study
260–1
innate in children 259
Lavater's drawings 193
muscular involvement
9, 29, 30
photographic record of
271, 276–81
recognition of 260–6,
268
regional differences 268
Epicanthic fold 37
Erasmus 5, 16
Erogenous zones
159–60
Erotic interest of face
159–61, 174, 175–6,
178
Eskimos 39, 41, 48
European,
cosmetic fashions
65–79
scarification 52, 54
tattooing 58, 59
wigs 86–91
Evolution 2, 3–4
Excitement evident in
eyes 263
Eye,
and beauty 142, 143,
144, 145, 146
change in ageing 23, 24
colour and character
217–18
colour and race 36, 37
contact and intimacy
263–4
cosmetic surgery 133–4
cosmetics 21, 48, 61,
63, 76, 77–8

emotion expressed in
263, 270
in folk legends and
symbolism 170, 172
male/female 21, 22
in physical illnesses
235, 236
in phsiognomy 197,
199, 202, 217, 229–
30, 271
squint 236
Eyebrows,
and beauty 143, 144,
146
cosmetic surgery 133–4
in physiognomy 199,
201, 202, 217–18,
229, 271
Eyelashes,
and beauty 144, 145
bitten in love making
159
Eyelids, drooping 236
Eye-shading, strong
sign of femininity
21

Face,
asymmetry 18
features see Eye, Hair,
Mouth etc
lift and rejuvenation
134–5
mix 240, 243–4
images of 174–9
signs of character
180–215, 216–29
symbolising whole body
172–6
types,
Hippocrates 233,
236–7
Kretschmer's theories
237–9, 243
preferred shape 174–8
Faces Test (Liggett)
226, 227
Facial movement,
effect on sex percep-
tion 23
Facialisers 26, 27, 266,
268, 275
Facies hippocratica
181, 232, 233
Fans and 'fan language'
117–18
Fan dictionary 117

Fatty tissue 8
Fear, expression of
261
Female,
artificial beard
(Egypt) 97
tattooing 57
Female/male
beauty 146–9
eye contact and judge-
ment 264
facial differences 21
fatty tissue 8
hair and head-dresses
21, 22, 23, 81
see also Wigs
skull 4–5
Femininity 81, 146
Fevers evident in face
235
Foetal head 1
Folk legends 170, 172
Forehead,
and beauty 143, 145
in physiognomy 199,
202, 206, 217, 219
Four basic tempera-
ments 184, 192
France,
cosmetics in 18th cen-
tury 69–71
head elongation 46
wigs 91
Freckles 68
Fucus 61, 68
Funeral masks 166

Gall, F.G., phrenolo-
gist 7, 205–6, 213
Galton, Sir Francis
243–4
Germany,
Nazi abuse of physiog-
nomy 231
sword scars esteemed
54
Gigantism (acrome-
galy) 235, 237, 238,
239
Glandular defects
evident in face 235
Glaucoma induced by
belladonna 23
Goitre evident in face
235
Golden section, golden
proportion 140

Greeks, ancient
  beards 97–8
  concept of beauty 140
  cosmetics 61, 63
  funeral masks 166
  hair 85
  *humours (tempera-
    ments)* 184–5
  tattooing 54
  physiognomy 181,
    184, 185
  wigs 90
  see also Mycaenae
Greeting customs 161

Hair,
  and beauty 142, 143,
    144, 145, 146
  chemical/dye treatment
    61, 85, 87, 88
  church attitude to 87
  *defects indicating
    glandular disorder* 235
  *in folk tales as symbol
    of strength* 173
  greying 23, 24
  lock as remembrance
    162
  male/female 21, 22,
    23, 81
  and race 35, 37
  removal at hairline 67,
    85
  style and treatment
    African 81
    *Greek, Roman,
    Egyptian* 61, 81,
    84, 85
    European,
    Mediaeval 66, 67, 85
    Cromwellian 87
    18th century 86, 88,
    89, 90
    modern 82, 83
    see also Wigs
Hare lip surgery 126
Hats 104–9
Head,
  of dead preserved
    162–3
  magic/sacred spirits in
    162, 163, 165
  shrinking 162, 163,
    165
  see also Skull
Head-dresses 104–9
Hippocrates, face and

health 181, 233, 236
  facial types 236, 237
Hypertelorism (Grieg's
  disease) corrected by
  cosmetic surgery 127

Identikit pictures 18
Illness,
  cure by medicine man
    166
  *mental, and facial
    features* 236–9, 243
  *physical, and facial
    features* 25, 233,
    236–7
Images of face 174–9
Imagines (Roman
  death mask) 182
Impressions, first 271
Indian,
  ancient cosmetic use 65
  caste tattooing 54
  early cosmetic surgery
    125
  veil 115
Indian, American
  fans (Iroquois)
    117–18
  features 33, 35, 221
  head of dead preserved
    163
  *head deformation as
    beauty* 46, 47
Individuality 18–19,
  131, 215
Indonesian tattoo 55
Inhibitions over
  cosmetic use 73, 76
Intelligence and facial
  features 5, 212, 219
Interfertility of races
  39
Internalisers 26, 266,
  268
Italian,
  masks 111
  personality 40, 41

Japanese,
  ancient,
  tattooing 54
  teeth filing 51
  modern,
  mouth tattooing 57
  racial features 37–8
  theatrical masks 169,
    171

Java masks 166, 168,
  169
Jaundice evident in
  face 235
Jaw surgery 132–3
'Jewish' nose 221
Jewellery, exploitation
  of 81
Judgement of person-
  ality,
  errors in 271–4
  halo effect 271
  intuition in 278–9
  *total configuration for
    successful* 18–19, 275

Kama Sutra 65
Kenyan wood carving
  174, 175, 176
Kohl 61, 63, 67, 68
Kretschmer, Ernst,
  facial types in
  psychiatric illness
  237–9
  in genius 243

Lavater, Johann
  Kaspar
  fame 188, 190–2
  *objective, love of man-
    kind* 192, 231
  physiognomy, theories,
    131, 181, 217, 218,
    219, 222–3
  *character interpreta-
    tions* 191–7, 215–21
  criticism of 201,
    204–5
  drawings of 193–5,
    202
Lead-based cosmetics
  67, 68, 88
Learning, phrenolo-
  gists' beliefs 213
Leonardo da Vinci,
  *drawings of facial
    proportions* 140
  grotesque heads 225
  nose important 131,
    228–9
Leptorrhine nasal
  features 35
Lie detectors 263
Liggett Faces Test
  226, 227
Lines of face 233
  see also Wrinkles

Lips,
  *distorted/pierced for
    beauty* 46, 48, 49
  *physiognomic signifi-
    cance* 198, 199, 202,
    222–3
  and race 38
  sexual signal 159
  surgery 133
  tattooing 56
Liver defects evident
  in face 234
Lorgnette 118
Love making, facial
  signals in 159–61
Lovers,
  *muscular movements in
    facial expression* 161,
    261–3, 264
  similarity of faces 201

Magic,
  in cosmetic use 64–5,
    67, 75
  of head and face 163
  mask enhancing 165
  tattoo enhancing 59
Male,
  cosmetic use,
  Greek, Roman 61, 63
  European 70, 73, 79,
    87
  fan use 117
  hair,
  Greek, Roman 85, 86,
    87
  Elizabethan 86, 87
  *see also Beards and
    Wigs*
  neck and chest dark 81
Male/female,
  beauty 146–9
  facial differences 21–3
  eye contact and
    judgment 264
  hair and head-dresses
    21, 22, 23, 81
  see also Wigs
  skulls 4–5
Marriage,
  *phrenology in choice of
    partner* 212
  and tattooing 56
Mascara 21, *see also*
  Kohl
Masculinity 81, 146

Masks,
death (Roman wax)
182
increasing magical
power 164
funeral 166
medicine man 166
origins 163
protective 111
theatrical 167–9
social uses 110–12,
114, 169, 170
versatility 169
Mediaeval,
beards 98
cosmetic surgery 122–5
cosmetics 67
hair 85
Medicine,
facial lines in 233–4
man 166
see also illnesses
Melancholia (depres-
sion) facial type 238
Melanesia, ear piercing
48, 49
Melanin 14, 36, 37
Meloplasty 134–5
Memories,
and beauty 152
factor in judgment
272
hair lock as 162
preserved heads as
162–3
Mental illness and face
type 236–9
Mesorrhine nose 30,
35, 43
Metaposcopy *see*
Physiognomy
Micronesia, tattooing
54
Military face 242, 245
Mitakuku 159
Mobility of face 7
male/female differences
in 23
cosmetics to conceal 23
in courtship 161,
261–3, 264
Mongolian features
30, 35, 43
Moon-like face
(Cushing's syn-
drome) 235, 236,
237

Moslems 116, 218
Mourning customs 97,
122, 162–3, 166, 182
Moustaches 101, 102,
103, 271
Mouth,
and beauty 143, 144,
145, 146
in folk legends 172–3
physiognomic implica-
tions 198, 222–3,
227, 271
surgery 133
see also Lips
Movement contrast 81
Movement in expres-
sion,
change with age 29, 31
of facialisers/internal-
isers 26, 27, 266,
268, 275
of lovers 23, 161,
261–3, 264–5
continual, producing
permanent change 241
Mud packs 74, 75
Musician, phrenology
of 206
Musculature of face
7–12, 23
in expression see
Emotional expression
and Movement
Mycaenaen death
masks 166, 167

Naevi 126
Nakedness and facial
interest 159
Narcissism in choice of
friends, colleagues
155, 272
Nasal index (Topinard)
35
Neck 81, 199, 235
Negro,
facial features 30, 35,
37, 38, 161
head elongation for
beauty 46
ritual scarification 51,
52, 53
Negroid 35 *see Race*
Nervous control of
expression 260–1
Neurological disorders
evident in face 236

New Guinea beauty
51, 59
see also Papuans
New Zealand tattooing
54, 57
Nicaragua, tattooing of
slaves 55
Nigerian,
greeting 161
legends 170
'No' theatre 169
North African tribes
48, 116
North America,
beards 100, 103
masks 111
see also Indians,
American
Nose,
artists attaching impor-
tance to 129, 131, 221
and beauty 143, 144,
145, 146
in disease 234–5
physiognomic implica-
tions 196, 197, 199,
202, 215, 219, 220,
221, 227–8
piercing for beauty
48–9
rubbing of as greeting
161–2
sexual signal 159,
161, 228
shape basis for racial
classification (Topi-
nard) 36
in stories and mytho-
logy 171, 230
surgery 127, 130–2
Novels, characters in
274

Papuans, nose piercing
48
Patches,
as party political
symbols 122
Male 121
Roman 61
17th–18th century
120–3
Modern 123
Language of patches
122
Pepys, on wigs 91
on patches 121

Persians, ancient 35,
90, 182
Personality (character),
altered by mask 169
assessed by Liggett
Faces Test 226, 227
and beauty 151, 225–
6, 227
and cosmetic sugery
126–8, 136
and facial features see
Phrenology and Physio-
gnomy
and imagined defects 230
measurement problems
228, 229
and race 39–40
Philippine Islands
customs 114, 161
Philosophic concepts
of beauty 151, 155
Photofit picture 18
Photographic sequence
in expression 276–81
Phrenology (organo-
logy, cranioscopy)
7, 205–8
benefits derived from
213, 215
commercialisation
209–12
criticised by church 212
in job application 209
Physiognomy (podo-
scopy, metaposcopy)
ancient 181–2, 184,
185, 187
see also Aristotle and
Avicenna
astrology in 182–4,
186–7
Della Porta's theory
186
of features see Eye,
Mouth etc
Lavater's theory see
Lavater
in literature 185, 186,
187
and science 185, 187,
205, 215
see also Judgement of
personality
Platyrrhine nose 35
Plumpers 118
Podoscopy *see* Physiog-
nomy

Politics and patch wearing 122
Polynesian tattooing 54
Primitive man 2, 3, 12
Profession,
evidence of, in face 241–2
examples of 246–57
Galton's face-mix 240, 243–4
and Kretschmer's face types 243–4
see also Artist, Criminal, Military etc
Progeria 28
Psoralen, skin-darkening drug 14
Psychiatric illness,
benefit from phrenology 213, 215
facial features 229, 237
performance in Liggett's Faces Test 226–7
Psychology,
of beauty 142, 150
of facial defects and cosmetic surgery 126–7, 136, 230–1
Pumice, teeth whitening 61, 68
Puperissium 63
Purdah 115
Pyknic physique 243

Quizzing glass 118

Race,
criteria for classification 31
Biblical 31
Linnaeus (skin colour) 31
Topinard's criteria 35
Deniker's criteria 37
examples 30–7
facial features, variations 4, 31–8
interbreeding 39
personality/temperament 39–40
UNESCO *statement* 38–9, 39–40, 41
see also Caucasoid, Mongoloid, Negroid
Regency dress and

cosmetics 70
Religion,
masks/idols in 166
self torture and sacrifice 51–2
see also Biblical references, Church and Moslems
Resemblances 201
Revolutionary face type 243
Rhinoplasty 130, 132
Rhitidoplasty 134–5
Ritual practices 50, 51, 52, 53, 64,
see also Tattooing, Cicatrisation, Scarification
Romans,
cosmetic use 60, 61, 75
death masks (Imagines) 182
decorative patches 121
physiognomy 181, 182
wigs 90–1
Russia, beards in 99–100

Sacred significance of beard 98
Sacred significance of face, head and hair 160–3
Sacrifice by cosmetics 75
Saddle nose 234
Scarification 52, 53
Schizophrenic face (acc. to Kretschmer) 238–9
Schnouda 70
Science,
and cosmetics 75
and physiognomy 185, 187, 205, 215
Scientist's facial type (according to Kretschmer) 243
Scurvy evident in face 234
Sebaceous glands 12
Sexual signals,
in beauty 150–1
of cosmetics 76
in facial features 159–61, 172–3, 178, 228, 261–4
in tattooing 56

Shape of face 5, 21, 30, 31,
and beauty 140, 143, 144, 145, 146
see also Face type and Symmetry
Similarity of friends 272
Simmond's disease 235
Size contrast, exploitation of 81
Size of face 21
Skin colour,
and ageing 24–6
and adolescence 29
attitudes to 14–6
chemical bleaching 16
experimental change of 14, 16
factors producing 12, 14
and illness 234, 235
and racial group 31
stereotyping errors 273, 274
Skin texture 8, 12, 23
Skull,
asymmetry 16
babies' deformed for beauty 43, 44–7
and body size 4, 5
male/female 5
size and intelligence 5
unusual shapes 5, 6
Slave tattoo marks 55
Smiling 7, 266
Soap 61, 72
Social/cultural background,
and beauty 43, 46, 155
and emotional expression 266, 268
see also Ritual
Socrates 203, 221
South American tribes 46, 48, 49, 52, 163, 165
Spain, fan in 117
Spectacles 118, 119, 271
Spirits in face 59, 170
Spurzheim 7, 208, 213
Squint 236
Stereotyping 272–4, 278–9
Sucking pads 8, 23
Symmetry/asymmetry 17–18, 140

Tattooing 54–9, 65, 159
Taxes on beards 98
Teeth treatments for beauty 50, 51, 61, 68
Temperament,
and environment 41
and physiognomy 184–5, 186
and race 39–41
Thailand theatrical mask 169
Theatrical masks 167–9, 171
Tibet,
head of dead preserved 162
theatrical mask 169
Topinard 35, 228
Toupées 95
Trobriand Islanders 159, 162
Tunisian veil 116
Tutankhamun's tomb and funeral mask 63, 97, 166, 167

Ugliness 141
UNESCO Statement on Race 35–9, 39–40, 41

Veils 112–17
Venus of Willendorf 178, 179
Victorian cosmetics and beauty 70–3
Vitiligo 16

Wigs,
antipathy with beards 100
Egyptian, Greek, Roman, Persian 90–1
European,
18th century 86, 91
modern 94–6
powder tax 93
professions distinguished by 93
Witches 170
Wrinkles 8, 12, 23, 24–5, 199

Yashmak (veil) *see Burqua, Chadri* 116
Yellow ochre 63

Z-plasty 133

262